An Iceberg in Paradise

An Iceberg in Paradise

A Passage through Alzheimer's

Nancy Avery Dafoe

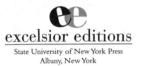

excelsior editions

State University of New York Press
Albany, New York

Cover art courtesy of Matthew Cincotta.

Published by State University of New York Press, Albany

© 2015 State University of New York

Excelsior Editions is an imprint of State University of New York Press

For information, contact State University of New York Press, Albany, NY
www.sunypress.edu

Production, Eileen Nizer
Marketing, Kate Seburyamo

Library of Congress Cataloging-in-Publication Data

Dafoe, Nancy Avery.
    An iceberg in paradise : a passage through Alzheimer's / Nancy Avery
Dafoe.
        pages cm
    Includes bibliographical references and index.
    ISBN 978-1-4384-5544-0 (pbk. : alk. paper)
    ISBN 978-1-4384-5545-7 (ebook)
    1. Avery, Phyllis—Mental health.   2. Alzheimer's disease—Patients—
United States—Biography. I. Title.
    RC523.2.D34 2015
    616.8'310092—dc23
    [B]   2014014917

10 9 8 7 6 5 4 3 2 1

This book is dedicated to
Phyllis Marie Unold Avery
and
Emerson Roy Avery Sr.

Contents

Illustrations

Foreword

Our brain offers us the capacity to self-reflect through the clarity of consciousness. When this is lost, we are lost, and such is the devastation of Alzheimer's disease. With most any other disease, even those that are progressive and inevitably fatal, as with some cancers or motor disorders, we can execute some measure of control through strength of mind. We choose a strategy of action to fight the disease, adopt an attitude, look back on the joys and sorrows of our lives, and plan how to live our last days. But with Alzheimer's, as the disease progresses our awareness fades, and the very patchwork of personality fractures, leading to behaviors and moods that are unexpected and uncharacteristic. We lose our capacity to cope and even lose the ability to express the fears and frustrations that beset us as our grasp of reality becomes ever more precarious. In short, we become helpless—and finally don't even realize it.

And so, with Alzheimer's disease, more so than with any other disease, it is up to others to provide the person with comforts, supports, and the overall logistics of living. The front line of these supports is usually given by the family. As poignantly expressed by Dafoe, the journey of care by family can be permeated with the landmines of guilt, misunderstandings, embarrassments, and frustrations. But it need not be such a perilous journey. We may grieve, but we shouldn't have to despair.

There is no cure for Alzheimer's disease as of this writing. Indeed, the past two decades have seen a string of profound disappointments in the medical field in this area. Pharmacological supports such as Namenda and Aricept have only mildly delayed the inevitable progressive symptoms of Alzheimer's, and hopeful new medications have proven to be false leads time and time again. Against this backdrop of failure, many doctors feel a sense of helplessness when treating a patient. "There is nothing we can do" seems the implied, if not overt, attitude. And yet there is everything we can do! The treatment of every disease, every condition, has two parts: the clinical side involves medical interventions and strategies designed to relieve the symptoms. But the other side, our attitude (and society's attitude) toward the disease is just as vital. We are, to some extent, as incapacitated and "sick" as others allow and perceive us to be, and it is here that we can do so much to help those with Alzheimer's.

If your spine is broken and you require a wheelchair, your condition is far better now than it was in 1920. You are, in a sense, far less disabled today. Why is that? Certainly not because we can now medically fix a broken spine or that people today with broken spines have superior physical movement. It is because our culture has progressively accepted and supported people who cannot walk, and this acceptance has, in turn, enhanced the quality of life for anyone requiring a wheelchair. There is little if any anger when someone in a wheelchair is first to board a plane or is entitled to a parking space close to a business. But what happens when a person with Alzheimer's disease pushes to the front of a line when boarding a plane while yelling, "Get out of my way!"?

Society is more forgiving and understanding of physical disability than of cognitive disability. There are many reasons for this discrepancy in attitude. Among them is the primarily subconscious dynamic of rejecting in others what we most fear ourselves. Most, if not all of us, are more terrified of losing our minds than of losing our legs. It is not easy to work on accepting a disease in others that we are too frightened to consider having ourselves. Another reason why society is more accepting of physical disabilities than cognitive disabilities is because physical disabilities are far more clearly noticeable. How many of us even think of the possibility that the elderly person pushing to the front of the line might have Alzheimer's disease? Indeed, the invisibility of the decline of mental capacity fools even those closest to the person suffering from it, as Dafoe clearly illustrates with herself and her own family.

Unfortunately, even when Alzheimer's is recognized by family members, this insidious disease allows them to hide the condition from friends and acquaintances, often at great cost. Bad behavior is perceived as bad behavior, and the person exhibiting it must take ownership of those gestures and that language. The slow and hidden progress of Alzheimer's lends itself to a rejection of having it, and with that rejection, how can we move on to assure that others treat the sufferer with kindness?

Dafoe chronicles these misunderstandings and other perils of providing support for her mother while offering the reader the many ways we can better "treat" Alzheimer's disease. Most importantly, we are consistently reminded of her mother's humanity. Perhaps this is the most important lesson of all. We need to learn that a person with Alzheimer's is the sum total of everything he or she has been, not the product of current status. We are thus treated to the sum total of Phyllis Marie Avery.

She was a loving mother, a devoted wife, a dedicated teacher, a lover of books, a skilled journalist, an introspective thinker, a cook, a bridge player, and so much more.

We must accept when someone has Alzheimer's disease because we really have no choice, but, in so doing, we need to view it as a passage rather than an end product, and we should be open to its existence if we expect and ultimately demand that others support those who have it. There is not yet a "cure" for Alzheimer's disease, but there are many ways that we can make its passage one of dignity and respect. Its tragic consequences need not be compounded by our fear and ignorance but instead can be softened by our compassion and understanding.

Ralph Hesse
Psychologist

About the Author of the Foreword

Ralph Hesse currently teaches psychology at the State University of New York at Cortland and at Tompkins-Cortland Community College (TC3) in Dryden, New York. He is retired from his position as a psychologist at the Developmental Services Office in Cortland, New York. Hesse has facilitated a support group for individuals who are caregivers for persons with Alzheimer's disease, doing so for the previous six years at Walden Place, an assisted living facility, in Cortland, New York.

Acknowledgments

Hesitating before committing this personal narrative to paper, I considered Vladimir Nabokov's words in his autobiography *Speak, Memory*, in which he waited before writing in order, "to avoid hurting the living or distressing the dead."[1] Part of me was profoundly reluctant to go back over that ground, return to some of the ugliness that accompanied the journey through my mother's illness and father's death as a result of Alzheimer's disease. When I began to experience the power of healing through writing and an honest look at the difficult circumstances, I finally made the decision to continue this project in hopes that I might help others who must make this journey.

I waited for a season after my mother's death before relating my book in poetry and prose because I wanted to preserve the secret my father worked so hard to protect. Not wanting to be disloyal to his impulse after their deaths any more than all the years that preceded their tragic ends, I pushed this story aside over and over until it would not rest.

We live with secrets, but I suspect this particular secret caused more harm than preserved good. We are always weighing the costs of our actions, and I have wrestled with this thorny burden for longer than I would have wished. In making the decision to complete this project, I am particularly grateful to my family, my daughters Colette and Nicole Dafoe, my husband Daniel Dafoe, and my son Blaise Dafoe.

A deep debt of gratitude is owed my professional reviewers: Ralph Hesse, who wrote the Foreword to *An Iceberg in Paradise*. In addition, my colleagues and friends Barbara Crossett, Cindy Hlywa, Jennifer Kirchoff, Bill Kirchoff, Amanda Smith, Maureen Watkins, and Keith Ward contributed to this final product through insightful readings and valuable commentary. Gratitude is also due Library Media Specialist Susan Padjen for her assistance. My sister-in-law Marilyn Avery and youngest brother Lawrence Avery were my earliest readers and encouraged me to continue the work.

Keith Ward was also instrumental in providing one of the first audiences for *An Iceberg in Paradise*, excerpts from which were read at the Last Stand event held in the spring of 2013 in the auditorium of ESM Central High School in East Syracuse, New York.

I would also like to acknowledge my siblings who each traveled through this difficult passage: Lawrence Avery, Dianne Avery, Phyllis Ann Avery, Robert Avery, and Emerson Avery Jr., who passed away during the time of our mother's illness and after our father's death.

Poetry Acknowledgments

The author's poem "Memory" first appeared in print under the title "According to Nabokov," in Gypsy Daughter's literary magazine *Brown Bagazine*, issue 10, 2010. "Lantern as Moon" was first published by the New York State English Council in volume 64, number 1, of the 2014 winter issue of *The English Record.* "Before I Knew My Father" was included in volume 25, 2011 of the twenty-fifth anniversary commemorative issue of the *Comstock Review.* "Composed on a Napkin" was read in San Francisco's Koret Auditorium, and won first place in the Soul Making Literary competition. All poems are the original work of the author.

A Note on the Title

Although icebergs in Paradise Bay, Antarctica is a geographic phrase indicating a location, the image created by the words "icebergs in paradise" has been widely attributed to Vladimir Nabokov, appearing in his novel Lolita.[1] My title is drawn indirectly from this work, as well as from a quotation by Orhan Pamuk in his book Other Colors, specifically his essay "Cruelty, Beauty, and Time: On Nabokov's Ada and Lolita," in which he compares icebergs to memory.[2]

After the Fall

Memory,
according to Nabokov—
for all its beauty and cruelty—
is an iceberg in paradise, the
metaphor staying with me as
I left my mother with her head
tilted too far back, her still beautiful
brown eyes open too wide,
behind them an iceberg had
already been cut adrift, pulled
from the orientation of land mass,
floating with its rich bluish-white
recollections entombed now on
open, cold seas, and the only
comfort I took away was that
she didn't seem to notice
drowning.

On March 21, 2005, at 8:25 in the morning, my father Emerson R. Avery Sr. died following a fall that occurred a month earlier in the predawn hours of February 17. In those dark hours in

February, he lay at the base of the stairs, alone, in pain, and drifting in and out of consciousness. My mother was walking down their street in the snow, wearing only her nightgown. She had left her house again, not recognizing it as her home. Sometime after seeing her outside, a neighbor called and an ambulance arrived. I'm sure that they did not expect to find my father lying unconscious at the bottom of the basement stairs, one tragedy compounded by another.

Indelibly, I know the very night he tumbled onto the hard concrete and the date he finally succumbed weeks after that cataclysmic fall. What I don't know with any certainty is how he came to be standing at the top of the stairs in the middle of the night when he was exhausted after a hectic workday; he was a normally sound sleeper. I believe, however, that my mother's Alzheimer's had something to do with it.

A practicing, highly regarded attorney, Emerson Sr. was balancing caring for my ailing mother with his legal work schedule and his recovery from a stroke a few years before. He didn't find much rest at work or at home, but he did not want to accept help either. Being fiercely independent and proud of it, Dad must have believed that through strength of character he could overcome almost any trial.

I can only speculate, however, that my mother's illness had played a role in why he teetered then fell down from that top step. One side of Dad's body was slow to react after the stroke he had suffered, but that did not explain why he was standing at the point of exit in the middle of the night.

This vision of my father at the bottom of the steps continues to paralyze me with horror. Occasionally I wake in the morning to this unsettling backdrop resting in my brain like a surreal canvas before me. Then I think of my mother walking out by herself into the dark, early morning.

The call came while I was teaching, and I had to turn to my class and force myself to focus them on a task as I grappled with comprehension. You are never prepared for those calls, I realized. Dad had looked great the night before, I kept thinking, remembering my visit to my parents' house in town. In fact, he seemed a good ten years younger than his chronological age, coming home from his Florida trip tanned and looking fit. After picking up Dad at the airport and dropping him off at his house, I decided to head home to check on my teenage son rather than go out to dinner with my parents, as Dad had suggested, a decision I returned to again and again with torturing regret.

Trying to absorb the words over the phone, my typically chatty group of students was suddenly silent, as if the world had ceased moving on its axis. Everything stopped for an instant, even my brain. I had crossed into that other realm, the one we scarcely notice when situations are generally going right for us, but the place where T. S. Eliot's *Unreal Cities* loom. I had entered that unnatural place, the one that moves us in parallel direction.

When I stood in the hospital emergency room—with my sister-in-law—looking at my father's astonishingly swollen, bruised, and bloodied face, I could not believe what had happened. Dad was sitting up and conscious but unable to talk, tubes running down his throat. He shook his head slowly as if he perceived the shame of it, not the pain. He looked as if he wanted to tell me something, but it was too much effort. At first, I tried to read his eyes—significantly narrowed by swelling—but then I told him that we could figure it out later. I thought we would have occasions for those conversations. We never did. That scene turned the clock back again and again as I tried to make progress.

Stopping all productive actions and intellectual absorptions for an instant, I sat in my living room in the warm leather chair near the fire, closed the pages of a book, and listened. The suddenly loud ticking of the wall clock became a trigger to another era when I was young, an inconsequential child lying in that spare room in my grandparents' house, filled with old clothes, boxes of other lives; my sister and brothers had already fallen asleep, their movements detectable as dreaming, and I experienced more than heard the clock ticking, felt its thumping with my beating heart.

Even as a child, I was aware of this reminder of our temporal existence, and much more, of the approach of losses to come, of an unidentifiable sadness, of the essentially lonely nature of being human even in a room inhabited by people you love. In my own house, in that instant of recognizing the motion of the clock, I returned from childhood not to the living room of my home as an adult but to the point in time of my father's struggle to survive.

Finally returned in temporal space to my living room— with so much of the focus on my dad, who was fighting for his life—I needed to immediately turn my attention to my mother, because her primary caregiver was hospitalized. In those weeks between my father's fall and his eventual death, I was called out of class on a number of instances. Life was interrupted, or the interruptions became my life.

How had my father managed it all? I wondered. He never told me about the instances when he had to leave his law practice because of issues with my mother at home. Never complaining, he dealt with so many problems; I look back now and am amazed at his capacity to absorb those punishing emotional and physical blows.

Nothing but questions punctuated the air. When did Phyllis Marie Avery get Alzheimer's? There is no clear delineation as to when she first showed warnings of having this type of annihilating dementia. This is not unusual, as anyone dealing with Alzheimer's disease (AD) will attest to because the onset may occur as early as ten to twenty years before the pronounced indications of severe memory loss, according to U.S. National Institutes on Health.[1]

Who keeps track of the minutia of the lapsed, filing it away until the instant when such odd records must be retrieved from the brain, deciphering fifteen years later the date a loved one first lost a wallet, a pair of earrings? And if we began keeping such awful accounts, we would certainly live in a state of constant paranoia. Everyone forgets his or her keys at some point, I reasoned, or perhaps, rationalized. What separates the occasional lapse from foreshadowing?

What I do know is that the struggle resulting from this affliction within our family and the tension between my parents—to say nothing of the desperate battle going on inside my mother's head—was so secret and tortured that it is only after I've had seasons to reflect on and revisit incidents, restoried how I acted, spoke, and appraised situations during my mother's protracted battle with Alzheimer's that I wish I could have helped more, proceeded in another manner, reacted better in some way. I know that the toll taken on our family was monumental.

Looking back with recall intact, I am also aware of the fact that individual members of my family will have experienced or remembered contrasting versions of the same events because our perceptions are—to varying degrees—subjective. Memory, in all of us, is an imperfect arbiter, but it is also our most powerful connection to each other and our former lives. Who would any of us be without our memories? And this insidious disease takes that which is most precious.

Looking back, I am equally certain that my father's devotion to my mother was absolute, that his unequivocal love and loyalty to her was emotionally costly and excruciating for him, and that we all could have handled my mother's Alzheimer's better—perhaps helped her more, helped each other more—if only we had better understood and accepted this silent, cruel intruder in their house.

This is not a medical text about transporter proteins and movement from blood to cerebrospinal fluid, about the death of neurons; neither is it a clinical book about psychological aspects associated with Alzheimer's, nor the science and psychology of illness. Rather, this book is about a passage.

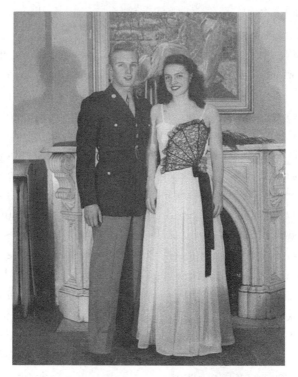

Figure 1. Phyllis Marie Unold and Emerson Roy Avery Sr. are shown in this photo taken shortly after the end of World War II, at what might have been their wedding but was instead a formal dance where their courtship and long journey together began.

At its center is a tribute to my mother and father, their love for each other and how we look at someone with Alzheimer's, how we behave in the presence of people who have this disease. It is also about our human connections, loss, and holding on until there is nothing tangible left to hold.

One of the reasons that Alzheimer's is so onerous for people to manage in caregiving is that the emotional states we take for granted, as a means of expressing how we are feeling, seem to float adrift, like those lonely icebergs addressed by Nabokov.

When I first saw a photograph of an iceberg floating, with the greatest proportion of its mass below the surface, I knew that was the image I wanted to accompany this story. The iceberg with its mass below the surface suggested all that remained hidden or lost. That loss creates confusion not only for the person with Alzheimer's but for the caregivers, as well.

The last clear statements that my mother made when she was able to articulate her wishes—before her confusion became such that her most immediate desires and conscious thoughts were taken from her through the death of brain cells—was that she not be placed in a nursing home, and, paradoxically, that she not become burdensome to her family; that she live the rest of her life with the dignity she had worked so hard to carve out. It was, however, as if her wishes threw her life in reverse and offered only the promise of each inversion. It was in trying to honor those wishes that my father met with such profound difficulty in caring for my mother.

Rather than try to bury the anguish of having had a mother with Alzheimer's and the circumstances of her final days, as well as those last days of my father's, I have chosen to remember it all to the extent that I am able and relive as much of it as I am capable of in order to look at this period in our lives clearly.

My mother's Alzheimer's disease held tyranny over us for a very long period of time. James Joyce wrote, "[s]ecrets, silent, stony sit in the dark palaces of both our hearts: secrets weary of their tyranny: tyrants willing to be dethroned," in his novel *Ulysses.*[2] I thought of this quotation when reflecting on my mother's disease. It was not Phyllis's domination, after all, but that of an unseen, silent manipulator—the disease itself, and AD made us look at Phyllis Marie differently.

When the picture of my mother, when the memory of my father's eyes, would not let me leave this behind, I returned to the whiteness of the blank page and began writing. I realized that the dynamics of the disease remain a mystery, yet other aspects have become clearer as the emotional charges accompanying events receded after an interlude; Alzheimer's robs memories in the person who has it and appears to cause distortion of memories in family members recalling emotionally difficult events involving the person with the disease. There are snippets of our conversations floating in the ether, as conceived by the ancients. Yet, none of us are immune to imperfections in our catalog of life's events. Mine are as subjective as the next person's, but they are sharpened by the habits of writing and by the architecture of a careful observer.

Not long ago, I had a conversation with our school resource officer who was discussing why he preferred to look at tire tracks, the pattern of broken glass, and other physical evidence at an accident site rather than listen to eyewitness accounts of what each person recollected. He stated that if he asked five people to give an account of the accident, he would receive five conflicting versions of the event.

This cautionary anecdote reminded me that my version of events—my recall of this passage, my "truth"—is perhaps no more accurate than a conflicting story by one of my siblings or by my parents' friends. I wanted, however, to attempt to learn from this tormenting experience of her disease that stole so much from her, from all of us. Memory is an imperfect construct from which we learn or unlearn, but it is also necessary in the process of discovering what makes us human. This ability to trace back is tied to perception and how we interpret a whole cornucopia of stimuli. It may be the most important of all human faculties.

A whole spectrum of responses is possible when we consider how individuals envision from mimetic power. Perhaps because I am continuing to work through those responses and because understanding the journey might help others trying to navigate this arduous course, I have chosen to write this book. It remains a choice that will affect other people—specifically my siblings—but a decision with results that I hope they will find solace in, or at least understanding of how the events in some ways shaped our lives but did not define any of us.

This book is about a passage through a devastating illness, but I hope that my words speak to my parents' extraordinary love and devotion to each other and my love for them.

After my father died and my mother was living in an assisted living facility, I went through their house to pack away their former lives. Each item I held was experienced like an unexpected, dreadful jolt, but I stopped when I came to her electric typewriter. Rolled on the table and fallen to the floor in their study was a long scroll of paper on which she was composing. Phyllis was writing a book about teaching elementary school children, a book in which she offered helpful suggestions for parents. In the middle of a chapter, in the middle of a sentence, the words stopped, cut off.

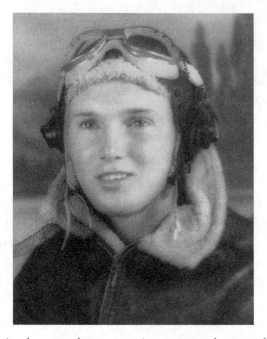

Figure 2. At the age when many American students graduate from high school, my father was flying over Africa during World War II.

I read and reread them and discovered the repetition of sentences, even whole chapters, that was increasingly apparent as I continued through the book. Prior to the manifestation of the disease, Mom must have known that matter and relationships were disappearing. The surface of her life was changing shape in a way that she could neither predict nor prevent. Somehow, she didn't dare tell anyone, or at least anyone other than my father.

The design of this book is intended to mimic the way memory works with new details emerging as we go back over incidents. The book expresses a personal journey in poetry and prose, dedicated to my parents, but one in which caregivers and relatives of a person suffering from Alzheimer's may find help, comfort, or recognition in dealing with AD in their families. Because it is not easy to talk or write about, this harrowing odyssey found its way into my poetry without my conscious effort at first. As intervals passed, I saw the emerging patterns and recognized a desire to create beauty from so much ugliness and pain.

Why bring poetry into a text about dealing with Alzheimer's in the family? There were spells when the pressures and bleakness of this annihilating debility in our family were nearly unbearable. Poetry permitted a bridge between what is spoken and unspoken and between what is consciously surmised and what remains untranslatable. Writing poetry and sharing it with others who are struggling with this disorder in their families has become a way for me to fight against that horror, offering words that transcended what my parents and our family went through, offering some consolation when my parents' world seemed permanently fractured or disfigured.

My sister-in-law recently shared with me the fact that she has been writing poetry as a way of dealing with the loss of my brother and her husband. He died too young, and she began to write creatively in order to deal with that seeming unimaginable reality. We often talk about the paradoxical healing power of creating a poem that is centered in the heart of pain.

I wrote the poems before the nonfiction text in which they are interwoven, however, and I recognized that they contained the emotional core, quietly directing the prose that followed the other aspects of the journey through this hostile foreign land. Writing poetry about these experiences somehow transformed them for me, allowing me to talk about my mother, my feelings about her illness, and about the cryptic conversations we were forced to have with others, as well as each other, because of this unstated promise not to confront this awful ailment head on. While not every poem will speak to every person who travels this difficult road, it is my hope that each one will offer something different to individuals who might not have made such a connection otherwise. ■

Chapter One

Uncertainty

Diving into the Unknown

On either side of narrow line
on which you walk, run, or drive along,
there is acute disappearance of all
that is known, and you're reminded
of a fresco painting from
The Tomb of The Diver in Paestum,
once the Greek City of Poseidonia,
where a young man,
not unlike your son, at least in age,
may be seen perpetually leaping from
formidable, rough stone walls
into uncharted seas,
his head held high as he stares
straight into light-blue waters,
the dropping off like looking out
over mountain roads—nothing to stop
a precipitous descent.
But you hug an imaginary line
as if it is the last entity
you will embrace.

For a long time—during the period of my mother's illness—I felt uncertain of nearly everything. That tension produced by these questions—What was wrong? Why was it happening?—was almost unbearable. Like my father, I refused to accept the evidence in front of my eyes, evidence that suggested there was no logical explanation and no cure. The mother I knew was not returning.

There is a haunting poem by Howard Nemerov titled "The Human Condition," in which a man waits in a motel room wherein he, "pace[s] the day in doubt / Between my looking in and looking out,"[1] the uncertainty of his ambivalent condition agonizingly transparent. The man exists in a domain—or between these expanses—of which he is unsure, the reality and unreality. This feels like the domain of experiencing Alzheimer's. For me, it was as if I was trapped and waiting for someone or something.

There is an awful, uncertain air that AD sufferers inhabit for part of their lives near the end, and it is intermittently the realm entered into by family members of those suffering from Alzheimer's. Unlike the certainty I feel about my father's tragic fall and death, there was little certainty about my mother's terrible malady.

I could not write the title of this chapter without thinking about numerous works of literature in which uncertainty is a theme, perhaps because the concept points so accurately to our human existence. Uncertainty is particularly fitting terrain for those dealing with Alzheimer's because that ground keeps moving from under us. All of those touchstones defined by memory begin first to appear opaque, and we are unnerved before they disappear altogether for the person suffering from this disease.

After I discovered that my mother had Alzheimer's, I found myself wondering what she knew or didn't know during that period in which bewilderment was the starting point in a daily battle. She masked her confusion as best she could. It was only later, when we began to find items in strange places that our questions started to multiply. A glove in a shoe, a sock in a box of cereal—no item was too strange, no location too weird in terms of places common items were discovered.

She also began throwing away items of value, some of which we never recovered, finding out too late that she had tossed a necklace or a ring away. Initially, it must have caused her agonizing stress to realize that she did not know where items were, at points even what the objects represented. Far more disconcerting, however, are the misplaced emotions, substituting what appeared to be anger for some other more appropriate affect. Frustration and confusion deeply held look like anger, and it seemed to be the place she fell into when her fear was most deeply rooted.

On a distant Saturday afternoon, I arrived at my parents' home with a bag of cookies purchased from a local bakery. At that point, my father was struggling for his life in the hospital, slipping in and out of consciousness and unable to talk. My mother was wandering in their rather massive house with a home health care aide nervously watching her movements.

The cookies were my mom's favorite kind, but when I offered them to her, she took the bag and threw it at me, cookies flung out across the kitchen, a broken piece hitting me in the cheek. Initially, I was upset with her for her irrationality. Already exhausted (I had just come from the hospital and was more worried about my father at that particular juncture), I wondered how much more I could take. Of course, I would learn that I had to take so much more. Only later, did I try to go back and consider what might have triggered her peculiar response. I knew so little about Alzheimer's then.

When it comes to Alzheimer's, certainties are still few. Even the estimate of the number of people with this type of dementia's diagnosis varies, with National Institute on Aging's statistics suggesting upward of 5.1 million Americans currently affected with Alzheimer's.[2] This site states that, "unless the disease can be effectively treated or prevented, the number of people with it will increase significantly if current population trends continue."[3] That is, indeed, a frightening pronouncement.

The nature of the disorder makes for the predicament of dealing with it by families and even medical practitioners. It was a surprise for me to learn through personal experience that this type of dementia is infrequently diagnosed early. It is particularly difficult to consider this type of memory loss in a loved one, and it is often easier to come up with alternative explanations for odd actions, misplaced items, and examples of memory loss and confusion.

Although physicians know the proper medications to pre-scribe to manage the psychotic episodes associated with this disease, it is not really their job to manage the emotional fallout of this diagnosis, and that burden falls to the most immediate caregivers. While there are health care professionals prepared to help families, as well as the person with Alzheimer's, the family first has to seek out those professionals, know where to go and what to ask. Yet some of the best ways of coping with AD in the family appear to be counterintuitive, but it is up to the patient's families to advocate for their loved ones and themselves. Neither my father nor I knew how to go about being advocates for my mother or for the type of care she needed. It took us far too long to get to that point.

"Your mother had an accident."

"What? Is she okay?" I looked around the room and saw Mom standing near the doorway. She appeared to be fine, except she looked suspiciously at us.

Dad nodded his head but in a way that indicated nothing was fine. "She hit a woman with kids in her car."

Mom turned with an angry expression on her face. "I did not hit her. She hit me."

"She hit your car? Where?"

"She ran right into me. Driving like a crazy person."

"Was she ticketed?"

"I didn't get a ticket!"

"Nobody was ticketed," said Emerson Sr. I still do not know if my father was telling me the truth in that situation. He was far more concerned with my mother's feelings than the collision of vehicles.

"The policeman said it was that woman's fault." Mom was becoming increasingly agitated and yelling at that point.

"No," said Dad, shaking his head with sorrow rather than disagreement. "No, he didn't, Phyllis."

"Don't you tell me; you weren't there!" At that point, Mom's voice was strained, nearly hysterical. She was almost shaking with what appeared to be anger.

"Mom, don't worry about it. It's over, and you're not hurt. She wasn't hurt; the kids and their mother weren't hurt, right?"

"They could have been," said my father.

"Don't you say that," yelled Phyllis Marie, walking out of the room and then turning around and standing there near the doorway.

"Dad, you can't let her drive anymore," I almost whispered.

"I can't," said Dad.

"Hide her keys," I suggested.

"I can't do that to her," he said, looking defeated.

Eventually, my father did hide my mother's keys, but it was not really necessary since she was beyond the ability to recall what to do with them even if or when she came across a set of car keys. I watched her take house keys and try to open the door of her car one afternoon.

Years before we recognized her condition, she had begun exhorting a promise from my father to never put her in a nursing home. She had an irrational fear of nursing homes based on misconceptions. I wonder now whether or not she was already experiencing early manifestations of the disease at that particular point? I suspect that she was, that the fear was driving her angry demand.

Recurrently, when my husband and I were in the front seats driving my parents to an event, my mother would lean over to my father and whisper conspiratorially, implying that my husband and I wanted to get rid of her, to put her in a home. We could barely hear her, but we always heard my father say, "I'll never let them do that to you." And he kept his promise, while he was alive.

It was only years later that I saw how helpful breaking that promise could have been. It might have saved my father's life. My mother's care in both the assisted living facility and the nursing home allowed her to be comfortable and her care well-managed, in a safe environment, far better than my father could create for her in their home once her disease progressed.

Of course, Dad's comment in the car was also hurtful to me, even though neither of them meant their words to be vexatious. Initially, I did not want my mother in a nursing home, either. If I could have had my preference, they would both be alive and living happily and independently. However, I also did not want them to be injured because they could not care for each other at home.

This dilemma is familiar to nearly everyone with aging parents, particularly those with some form of dementia, in some manner. Few people have the good fortune to remain completely independent their whole lives and die peacefully in their own beds.

Would all of the events and their consequences have been less tragic if my father had not been so protective of my mother and so vigilant in his promise to her? Even when I did not know what clock was ticking, I deduced the pressure of the inevitable, of tragic conditions weighing down on us. His secretiveness and morose qualities were particularly unsettling because my father had always carried an air of optimism about him. He was fighting with himself as well as with his wife. Then he felt he had to fight his children.

Phyllis had always been more of a realist than Emerson, but she was not as prescient as she tried to project. On several occasions, she declared that she was going to die young like her mother and father had. That early loss may have made her feel lonely and isolated even in a room filled with family. Increasingly, you could see it in her eyes—the fact that she was in the room with you and not in the room at all. Phyllis did not die young, however; she lived until she was nearly eighty-three.

I recall standing in the dining room at the assisted living facility where my mother stayed for three years after my father's death, and suddenly becoming aware of the detached threads of familiarity around me. What initially was discerned as an illness that alienates on so many levels—the mind from the body, the members of the family from one another, the debilitated person from family and friends, and the family dealing with Alzheimer's from the rest of the community—began to reveal itself as remarkably patterned.

Inadvertently at first, then deliberately, I heard the same conversations about various incidents in people's lives around me that my family had experienced with this pathosis as the silent, angry member. The irony is that most likely each of the individuals in those family groups presumed that he or she was going through this terrible battle in isolation. There were middle-aged daughters and sons speaking softly and then sharply to their aging parents, confused about what to make of their parent's lack of responses or inappropriate statements. There were the inevitable embarrassments as out of context comments punctuated the air, the insults that flowed like acid in a sour room. There was anguish, of course, but it was masked by so many other conflicting emotions.

Family members of those with Alzheimer's often look like they are sitting in a dark room alone although the common room full of people is brightly lit. The strangeness of it is that we don't recognize these isolating actions and circumstances right away or we simply have no appropriate manner in which to deal with the strangeness of the experience. Then again, with uncertainty at the heart of this, we are not really sure what we are seeing and how we are interpreting the odd gesture, the disconnected phrase, the random pair of knitting needles in your mother's purse that is ready to be passed through an airport scanner.

Because of the nature of the Alzheimer's, it is one that many families do not recognize immediately, and then commonly deny, simply cannot believe, making excuses for the early indications that are perhaps missed or misunderstood. That was our family. We covered for each other in a nearly subconscious, compensating process, and then separately in a predictable but emotionally crushing insularity.

Yet the uncertainty is most profound for those directly affected by this attack in which the boundaries between reality and other planes of existence are blurred beyond recognition. A separate compass of this altered state looks very similar to psychosis, as the dementia progresses, but, at first, it appears as simply discomforting as the looking in or looking out of a surrealist painting—like the experience Nemerov related in his poem "The Human Condition," in which he described a Magritte painting referred to earlier in this chapter.

For a lengthy period of time, I didn't know what I was dealing with and, even less, how to approach the problem. People with Alzheimer's look lost and sporadically afraid or angry—the two emotions increasingly conspicuous and oddly interchangeable. Whether subjective or not, most of us move within parameters that distinguish between past and present if not the future. But someone with advanced Alzheimer's disease can no longer make those distinctions.

More than once, I looked up to find my mother staring at the kitchen counter—rubbing a spot repeatedly. "What are you doing, Mom?" I was compelled to ask, even though it should have been clear that the action was symptomatic. She proceeded with a paradoxical, indifferent urgency.

"What?" she would ask, pulled back from this other place, annoyed or frightened of the implications of my seemingly innocuous question. "I've got too much to do," she would say almost angrily and then sigh at the same moment that I wondered what it was she had to do. If I didn't distract her again, she would return to rubbing the counter, and a line from Shakespeare's *Macbeth* popped into my head: "Out, damned spot!"[4] but, thank goodness, I never said it aloud.

Any discussion of Alzheimer's is going to be focused on loss and the state of angst caused by that loss, as well as the uncertainty. Yet the subject also demands that we consider the bounty of our memories before those losses. In the words of Nabokov in his autobiography *Speak, Memory*: "How small the cosmos . . . how paltry and puny in comparison to human consciousness, to a single individual recollection, and its expression in words!"[5] I would only add to his truthful, lyrical words that this constellation of bright spots from antecedents compels us, causes us to turn and look back in reflection, regardless of the visions we face.

Chapter Two

Why Now? Why My Family?

Vanishing

With its distinct black and candid markings—
like a fine, black-inked pen on white paper—
as well as its penetrating movements,
the Great Northern Loon suggests
symbolization, diving as it does repeatedly
beneath surface of the way we first see;
its name from Old Norse meaning lame,
but also lament: it is not surprising that we
feel the dispiritedness of its disconsolate cry
far from shore where diver vanishes,
plummeting deeper. Then it reappears
farther out, and we consider
hidden territories covered, terrors
encountered in unfamiliar descent
into aphotic waters in which we dream.

One of my students recently wrote an essay about the death of her grandmother from Alzheimer's disease. The first question she raised in writing was, Why my family? I anticipated a slight shudder of the kind of recognition I didn't want to experience. Only later, when I was able to look back and frame questions about this period in my life did I ask why Alzheimer's happened to my family, as well. It is the question almost everyone asks silently if not out loud when this disease crawls into our midst.

Alzheimer's was identified as early as 1907 by Alois Alzheimer, according to the Emory University's Alzheimer's Disease Research Center.[1] While health care professionals may know about the disease, general knowledge of it did not seem to find its way to laypersons for many years. But not everyone finds his or her way to a medical professional during times when these early signs of the disease appear. I began thinking about the people who were believed by their family members to be mentally ill, about those who committed suicide, about the people who wandered off in the middle of the night and died, and their families holding those secrets inside.

An unexpected revelation was to learn that many people who were patients in the Alzheimer's unit with my mother had come from a variety of segments of society and the workforce— college professors, business owners, cashiers, clerks; there appears to be no social or economic favoritism with AD. Alzheimer's is as likely to show up in a very bright person as in an individual who is less gifted intellectually. It is not the result of poverty or wealth like some illnesses that have causes linked to poor living conditions or excess of drugs and alcohol.

My mother never smoked or drank liquor or even imbibed in the occasional glass of wine with dinner. She was diagnosed with breast cancer when she was only fifty-two, but she conquered it inasmuch as she lived for nearly another thirty-one years. Although she was not brave about all circumstances, she was remarkable in facing her cancer with determination to beat it and keep her spirits high. She even talked about looking at wigs with me during her chemotherapy treatment, and she seldom complained about her cancer. Her courage and resolve during her cancer treatments were inspiring. Then she got Alzheimer's.

Ironically, she was able to talk bravely about her cancer and her fight with it, but the word *Alzheimer's* was never spoken by her. By the time we knew she had this type of dementia, she was beyond being able to reason or discuss it. She had grown increasingly secretive and suspicious and acted as if the medications we offered to her were poisons. The woman who swore by everything a doctor said for most of her life was suddenly averse to seeing even the most learned specialist.

I was not any better able to deal with her dementia. My father, as well, denied any changes for a long time, and we were like lost children entering this unnatural realm, looking around, trying to get our bearings. Worse yet was the silent statement of blame. With this disease, you look for blame where none exists.

The uncomfortable, untenable answer to why my family is that there is no answer yet available. The response to why this pathosis manifested itself when it did is that there is no definitive response. For my father who waited patiently for Phyllis to have awareness of him again—for her to remember him and their life together—the silence turned into a roar that must have erupted on that final night of his life. How the disease manifested to her, I cannot even imagine.

My mother was a healthy, very intelligent, creative woman whose lifestyle—which could be construed as careful and cautious if not conservative—seemed to offer no clues as to why she contracted this deadly robber of her memories, her personality, and finally her life. Although she lived in a city growing up, she spent her entire adult life in the country. We did not live near a nuclear power plant or obvious source of pollutions or contaminants. It would seem the environment had nothing to do with the onset of her disease.

The search for answers early on left us all frustrated and unhappy, but there was no systematic search, no sharing of information with medical professionals, the only ones equipped to provide the type of answers we were seeking. Alzheimer's wormed its way into all of our relationships with one another, paradoxically insulating us from each other and from our community during this period.

After searching multiple websites for information on the disease, I discovered that a favorite author of mine—Gabriel García Márquez, like my mother and like his memorable character Colonel Aureliano Buendia—was losing his memory and was believed to have Alzheimer's, according to his brother.[2] But, like so much information we collect, that is subject to various perspectives and even denial, this information has been refuted by other websites and other García Márquez family members. According to the head of the foundation created by Gabriel García Márquez, "I will not argue or comment on interpretations of Gabo's private affairs and health, but I assert there is no medical diagnosis of senile dementia," the director of the New Journalism Foundation, Jaime Abello, wrote."[3] Of course, I thought, even in the life of a celebrated author, Alzheimer's carries such stigma that it is difficult to admit to even by those continually in the public eye.

I wondered what García Márquez knew, what he sensed as the world began to appear in detached segments. Did he hold another novel inside that he could not access? Was he afraid of writing the same phrase over and over? I thought about this as I recalled the scroll of writing—unfinished—that fell from my mother's computer, her words frozen and incomplete.

There has continued to be speculation that Winston Churchill—one of my father's heroes—had Alzheimer's but perhaps, here again, no definitive answer on the pathology has been determined.[4] A favorite singer of my mother's—Perry Cuomo—is believed to have had AD, and former President Ronald Reagan and his friend and fellow actor Charlton Heston both died of complications from Alzheimer's.[5] I imagined the difficulty faced by Reagan's cabinet members who knew that something was terribly wrong with their commander in chief, but they could not be disrespectful. The renowned Irish writer Iris Murdoch—a favorite of mine—publically struggled with Alzheimer's, as did Peter Falk, or the man many Americans knew by his alter ego, Columbo.[6]

The list of well-known people who have died from AD is lengthy and includes, in addition to a president, U.S. senators, Olympians, chefs, professional baseball and football players, singers, opera stars, and human rights activists. Remarkably democratic, Alzheimer's appears to have no political, religious, or economic preferences. In probably most of the cases of the disease, each family has wondered, why? What triggered the onset of this disease?

There seems to be some correlation between a blow or blows to the head and the onset of dementia; however, there are obviously people who have been struck in the head who did not die from AD or suffer from another form of dementia. It would also seem that high and perpetual stress levels may be a potential trigger, but much more research needs to be done before this statement can be accurately made or predictive. Science may yet lead us to fully understand the triggers of this disease, but currently is not ready to pinpoint exactly why someone gets AD or—much more acutely noted—how to cure a person with Alzheimer's.

The hopeful aspect of this topic, however, is that progress is being made, and the discussions today will likely be very different ones in ten to twenty years. In the meantime, most of us are not very good at accepting the "no answer" or waiting for a pharmaceutical that is not yet ready, but we can open our eyes and look straight into it—whatever that is—because averting our gaze will not make it go away or make it easier to bear. Understanding how the disease progresses and what to expect with the stages actually make the untenable situations more manageable and may offer the slight solace of living with less regret and guilt.

Chapter Three

Secrets

Eyes of Women

Mirrors of beauty, grace, and burdens,
disembodied eyes can only be seen from above,
as if, indeed, the artist JR laid down his canvas
to challenge gods with these sundered
images on the back of a lens.

Women's eyes, indistinct in motion—see this rumbling,
dizzying journey along rails, one car after another—read
then weep in rhythmic union. In focus, out of focus—
seeing abstracted—these totems compel, propel,
ride in the wake of what it is to be human
on tracks across the back of our planet.

Phyllis Marie Unold Avery had beautiful, brown eyes that were
expressive and showed her strength of personality and fire for
life. Only at the very end did her eyes begin to cloud over and
register no urgency, no wants, and no interests. This contrast
was felt particularly acutely by me because Mom had always
been so passionate about everything, and her eyes reflected and

registered her intensity and intelligence, her wonders, her disgust, distain, and her fears.

For a prolonged sequence of events—and here is where uncertainty is pronounced, because how many years is a matter of speculation, which members of the family are trying to piece together—we did not know my mother had this affliction. Changes in her behaviors and personality, as well as her aphasia, amnesia, and eventually, alexia were gradual and interrupted by the familiar, so we made excuses, looked in other directions, even cast some blame on her "quirks of personality" because we did not know or understand what was happening to her.

I believe that my father knew before any of his adult children or grandchildren, but the prognosis was so terrible for him to recognize that he denied it even to himself. He became an expert at covering up these instances of her odd behaviors, making excuses, not revealing what happened. After the initial events, the stories began to trickle out—purses that were left behind and returned by friends or retrieved by my father from restaurants, missing checks, missing money, and, later, multiple indignities.

Reconsidering my interpretation of events from the vantage point of new knowledge, I am amazed at what we had overlooked, the ridiculous conclusions we came to, and the lack of sympathy I initially had for my mother. Even if not one of the manifestations of Alzheimer's, her paranoia might have made sense in that context alone.

There was a Thanksgiving dinner in which only a tiny Cornish game hen was found baking in an oven, the little bird meant to feed over twenty people. My initial reaction was to laugh bitterly and then realize what this ridiculous situation portended. Perhaps this circumstance would have been less strange if my mother had not made countless meals for our increasingly larger family, and she had always been a very good cook and organized planner. Saving the day, my sisters went out and purchased a turkey, and we prepared a dinner that my mother had previously taken such pride in creating for her family. She, however, seemed strangely indifferent to the fuss around her. If anything, she acted annoyed with all of us for interfering. What is also strange is that we didn't immediately recognize these obvious indicators of the disease.

What was I thinking then, I wonder now? Did I imagine that my mother suddenly didn't want to cook anymore and that she was giving us her message indirectly? It was not as if my mother's vocabulary was always strange, however, so these weird lapses just seemed to be anomalies at first, and my father provided excuses, and we must have wanted to believe them as much as he wanted us to accept these alternative versions of events.

Not so long ago, on a cool evening, during a family gathering with my younger sister and her family visiting from out of state, Mom started the laundry, and our eyes began to water. My sister rushed her young children out of the house as my father yelled at his wife, "What are you doing?" when he discovered that she had poured an entire bottle of Clorox in the washing machine without turning on the water. The caustic fumes scalded our ideas of her competence, but she had an excuse, told a story, as to why she had made this error. As was typical during this time—she became defensive and angry with us for showing her no compassion when she had made a "simple mistake."

Although it distresses me now, I believed then that these lapses and other oddities indicated that my mother was just getting forgetful, becoming meaner or stingier in her "old age." Why it did not occur to me that her actions made no sense, I can only imagine as perceptions clouded by emotion. We also had no knowledge of Alzheimer's disease.

I recall stopping by my parents' house to take my mother shopping, an activity that she used to love. When I picked her up, she seemed fine, but as soon as we began to walk around the store and aisles of dresses, she started blurting out rude statements, asking why we had come to a store with "old junk not worth buying." I took it as unfiltered honesty and hurried her out of the store—but Phyllis Marie could not really be hurried at that juncture of her illness—feeling embarrassed. Rather than cringe, I wish that I had quietly explained the situation to the store salesperson and allowed my mother to wander about and say whatever she wished. The truth is, however, it is not easy to manage people with AD.

Only much later did I realize that what she was experiencing and seeing in that store was very dissimilar from my perceptions. What exactly was the scene her brain produced? There is no way to discuss the manifestations of this disorder without addressing some of the ugliness and peculiarities. It changes the person you love, alters personality. Alzheimer's provided an alternate universe for my mother, and I was operating from another plane of existence.

In terms of my mother's physical appearance, she looked very much the same for many years, always younger than her chronological age. Her thick, brown hair and dark, expressive eyes remained distinctive features until nearly the end of her life. For years, there were few of the manifestations of other illnesses that encourage people to show pity or compassion. Her voice was strong; her vocabulary as expansive and sharp as ever, only now the words were running around out of context.

Alzheimer's, we discovered slowly, is not a type of brain impairment with immediate overt beacons—no gaping wounds, no sudden weight loss, and no loss of hair. Much worse, it is a sickness that robs the mind gradually, groups of neurons in

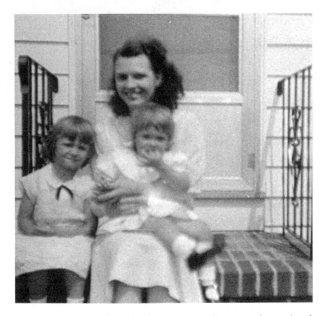

Figure 3. Our young mother Phyllis Marie is shown with me (on her lap) and my sister.

stages, and as such, the mind's normal responses. It is not a sickness that readily elicits sympathy or, certainly, empathy.

Alzheimer's alienates. Friends of my parents began avoiding seeing them; even some of their oldest friends stopped coming over. I was less aware of this initially, and only later did I ask my father why a particular friend did not seem to come around anymore. Dad always had reasonable excuses for his friends, as well. At some point, my mother had undoubtedly made what appeared to be a rude remark or remarks, and some people did not understand what was happening to her. They chose not to be uncomfortable.

My father might have received more sympathy and help if only he had not wanted to keep my mother's condition a secret.

I know now that he thought he was protecting her, yet the toll on both of them—on all of us—from harboring the unspoken was very great. It was entirely possible and reasonable to conclude that my father harbored her secret because she had kept silent about his stroke.

Seven years earlier, Emerson Sr. suffered a stroke. In spite of the problems it caused him, particularly during the recovery period, he did not want anyone to know about his debilities, and he went to work routinely. My mother spent exhaustive hours helping him improve his speech and changing their diets and lifestyle to help him regain ground he had lost. Her sole focus on my father during that period of recovery was extraordinary and fierce. She was protective even when no safeguards were necessary; in fact, she "protected" him from his children and grandchildren, even though we just wanted to help.

It was during that period when I suggested that Dad scale back his law practice and look for a smaller office with less overhead. Both of my parents did not want to hear these suggestions, however. Maintaining their independence and keeping as close to the routine as possible—to the lives they had lived together for so many years—became my father and mother's mission. In many respects, his resolve was admirable; it was also problematic for me because I was worried about him and about my mother, too, concerned when my mother had yet another car accident even though she was not injured, nervous about my father driving around because sensation in his foot had not been fully regained after his stroke.

The demands of meeting appearances were so great for them that I think they often forgot to eat. On multiple occasions, my parents showed up unexpectedly, late in the evening at my house. When they came in, Dad would always casually ask what we had for dinner, even though we had eaten hours earlier. I would fix them a quick meal, and they would eat and head home again, as if this turn of events was ordinary.

I believe that it was particularly formidable to tackle recognizing the auguries of my mother's illness because, initially, we were focused on not losing our father after his stroke. He had become the center of our attentions, and my mother began making needlessly cruel remarks to me that I took as some kind of Freudian competition. She accused me of taking articles from her, of not returning items I did not have.

Only now do I recognize the patterns and realize that they were not particularized to me. She was also sharp and rather mean to my brothers, particularly the eldest who lived in our town and who was dealing with his own grave illness. Many of her comments made no sense even then, but we construed other meanings, considered errors and misinterpretations as facts.

While riding with my parents around the lake on a warm summer afternoon, my mother began to criticize my brother whose own health was rapidly failing. Her accusations made no logical sense, but the more all of us tried to defend my brother and question her words, the more aggressive she became in verbally attacking him.

At last, my brother simply got up and walked to the front of the pontoon boat where he sat back down. As soon as my brother was out of her line of fire, she stopped talking angrily. I was so focused on protecting my brother that I failed to see the markers of illness in my mother, as well. I remember feeling tremendous anger that was stifled. I believed that my mother had to know what she was saying and the effect of her words.

When I look back now, I am amazed that all of us were so blind to the forewarning that now seems transparent, but the fact that each of us was taxed by these health crises in multiple ways partially explains our inability to clearly see what was in front of us.

Once during this exhausting period of time, I was driving to work when my attention was pulled from the road ahead of me and off to the side. There at the periphery, I witnessed a spectacle of turkey vultures whirling in a draft of warm air above the deer carcasses that had been buried in the median between roads. The vultures were gliding in sync as if in a coordinated dance, widening the arc of their movement at the top, resembling a living, feathered tornado with a single buzzard standing motionless at the center in this dark, slow fury.

The spectacle was arresting. It seemed like a portrait in madness, perhaps only because it was ugly and fascinating. I recall thinking that the strangeness of it was like being pulled into the world of the person with Alzheimer's, where nothing was the same and yet everything was the same, and the threat was at once imminent and imagined. I could not get beyond that terrifying sense of disquiet—that slow separation from the rational world—because I was also watching this ritualized dance between my parents simultaneously.

Chapter Four

Mistaken Identities

Mistaken Identities

Walking into the midst
of limitations,
of marriage,
he doesn't know how;
without apprehending,
she becomes a child
feeling sting of acrid words,
without full context,
followed by amplified silence
inundated with misery
as he travels the longest route
around the kitchen
and she slams drawers,
narrowly missing her fingers,
harshness hidden in
an unnatural diet of words,
providing clues without boundaries,
language—of sudden strangers—
falling like little stones.

Although my father had been in World War II, enlisting when he was sixteen and flying low over Africa and Italy, in the belly of a bomber when he was only seventeen years old, no event in his life had prepared him for his wife to mistake him for a stranger as they approached their fiftieth wedding anniversary. As hard as it was for her children and grandchildren, my mother's Alzheimer's was even more horribly tragic for my father. The affections that they shared had disappeared, and she replaced them with accusations, nonrecognitions, and denials. The greatest hurt, however, is that she did not seem to know him.

There is a curiously titled and apt book that comes to mind whenever I revisit a surreal scene set during the period in which we were dealing with my mother's infirmity. I bought the book because of the title alone: *The Man Who Mistook His Wife for a Hat and Other Clinical Tales*, by neurologist Oliver Sacks, offers stories in clinical psychology in which patients' brains cause even their sight to be altered. My mother made those strange mistakes in which she saw my father not as her husband but some stranger; she saw me as her mother, her sister, a neighbor, and sometimes as no one she knew at all.

In the Preface to his clinical narratives, Sacks wrote, "The patient's essential being is very relevant in the higher reaches of neurology, and in psychology; for here the patient's personhood is essentially involved, and the study of disease and of identity cannot be disjoined."[1] Disease and identity become comingled. As someone writing from outside the medical profession, that expression seemed to express what I felt happened to my mother; yet she was not her disease. It was, however, a Herculean trial not only for her but for the people around my mother to cope with her as she manifested this illness.

Only in retrospect was I able to fully recognize my mother's monumental struggle—and ultimately defeat—to try to retain her sense of self. Oliver Sacks quoted Ivy McKenzie in his "Part One: Losses, Introduction," regarding the ability to precisely define that struggle: "the human subject, striving to preserve its identity in adverse circumstances."[2] I would, however, change two words in McKenzie's description: *subject* and *its*. This was my mother striving to preserve who she was, where she had been, what she had known in the face of horrific, memory-robbing circumstances.

On the last night of his life as he had known it to be, my father came home to find his wife accusing him of trying to break into their house. I stood in their kitchen as he tried to convince her: "I'm your husband; don't you recognize me? Didn't you miss me?" It was as if her sight had been altered, too.

"You? I don't know you! Get out of here."

He persisted. "We've been married for . . ."

"I don't know who you are." Phyllis became increasingly agitated as Emerson tried to convince her of their relationship, remind her of their love. The argument appeared as if it went on for hours, but the tension was such that it probably lasted no more than twenty minutes or so. At last, she calmed down only after I made her a cup of tea, began agreeing with her, and my father was allowed to stay. I left them sitting together, thinking that they would be fine again.

In retrospect, the episodes that could be considered psychotic breaks were abundant, but we all tried so hard not to believe what we were seeing or hearing or that there would be a return to rationality. For a lingering period, too, my mother was able to have very normal sounding conversations around these episodic periods of misidentification of people and places. She might use just the right word, the most sophisticated word for the situation, and I could not conceive that she had any type of brain disease. How could she still access such vocabulary at will? How could her mind seem to work so well in some areas?

What was even more puzzling was the seeming fact that she was more likely to misidentify her husband or her daughter—the two people whom she saw habitually—than people she only occasionally saw. More than one of her acquaintances reminded me that, "Your mother seems fine. She knew me!"

A year after she was so delusional that she never knew or used my name and confused me with either real or imagined people from her past, she recognized her seldom seen son-in-law at her husband's funeral. She had not seen him in quite some time because my sister and her husband live in another state, but his name tumbled out as soon as she saw him. This was at the same funeral where she stated that either her uncle or her cousin had died. Yet, Emerson Sr. lay in the casket my sister-in-law and I had chosen. During that period, my mother could not even identify her husband much less make choices about caskets and gravestones.

For at least a couple of years before my father's death, my mother began to misidentify the city in which she lived. At first, she could be corrected and seemed to accept it, but later, she would not move from her confused position, becoming increasingly agitated.

During an afternoon visit, she told me that all of the women in their city had moved south. There were simply no more women in our area, she stated. The harder I tried to point out this obvious, ridiculous error, the angrier and more stubborn she became about defending her perception. She argued with passion and multiple points to support her confusion, appraised as an exercise in reasoned madness.

Before she was admitted to the assisted living facility, my mother mistook her own grandchildren for robbers on more than one occasion. Her house became a school, the bathtub mistaken for a toilet. While these incidents sound implausible, those mistaken identities became her daily existence and the challenges my father faced with her. Although I wondered what was going through her head, I had the more immediate concern of what she would do next. She had become increasingly suspicious as the people near her must have been taking on sinister and surreal qualities. Of course, as everything became fragmentary for her, we would have appeared malevolent.

When it comes to human dignity, we all count on our bodies not to betray us, but most of all, we count on our brains continuing to function as before. Yet, betrayal is what you get with this disease. Dad came to me on a number of occasions because he did not know what to do when Mom had soiled herself. At first, I could not believe it. My mother was one of the cleanest individuals I have known, and she was meticulous about her person and other facets of her life, including her dress and her house.

I recall trying to change my mother after a particularly depressing but vivid incident, and she seemingly became incredibly angry with me. "What are you doing?" she yelled. Trying to explain that I was removing her soiled pants, I realized that she was hitting me.

When she saw the wet clothing, she said, "I don't know whom those belong to. They're not mine. Did you put them there?" She did not recognize her own body functioning in the way it was. In fact, this display repeated itself numerous times, and she continued to be surprised as well as indignant about the situation. It was as if someone had tricked her by putting soiled apparel on her body.

I think that the nonrecognition of bodily functions was horrific for my mother, even in her confused state. For my father, it was mortifying and sad almost beyond comprehension. It almost paralyzed him from action.

Strangely, she had moments in which she seemed to be functioning as if she knew what was going on around her. I remember feeling very nervous when the assisted living facility's nurse came to her house to do an assessment because I was afraid that Mom would appear too coherent to be admitted to their Alzheimer's unit. What would we do then? During the first few questions of the interview, Phyllis was suspicious of her guest but polite and atypically appropriate in all of her responses. She acted annoyed with the questions rather than angry, but after several minutes, her defenses began to break down, and her answers became less reasonable. It was as if she was willing herself to pass the test, then lost her strength.

Waking up in the middle of the night, she must have reached out reflexively and touched the stand with the antique lamp next to her beautiful cherry bed and it was unfamiliar, and then she would have turned her head to the side only to see an old man with wild white hair matted near his temples. She would fix her desperate eyes on his gaping mouth, the point of origin of the snoring, actually his interrupted gasping, gulping breaths—the noise that woke her from a quieter place to this unknown bed in a foreign house. And she was terrified.

Then she would conjure up only the fears of a child, the sensations of a child, a lost child, one without even the comfort of a mother, and she would get up quickly and quietly, anxious not to wake the snoring stranger. In the dark, she would put on her tan, boiled wool hat but not her shoes, her socks already on because her feet were always cold in the winter, and she would wander through alien rooms in a crescendoing panic until she stumbled on a door, and with determination not to let them get her, she would step out into the snow, surprised that they had not bothered even to clean the sidewalks. Over and over again, someone brought her home.

This pattern of disquietude and confusion would be repeated for her until, finally, there were no points of exit.

Recently, while reading a book by the Turkish novelist Orhan Pamuk, I was struck by his lines at the end of *Silent House*, which spoke to this dread not only in people who had become lost in Alzheimer's but to all who have discerned themselves to be lost at some point in their lives: "If a person can live in the same house for seventy years and still be confused, then this thing that we call life, and imagine we have used up, must be such a strange and incomprehensible thing that no one can even know what their own life is."[3]

There were times near the end of that period when my mother was living at home when I thought it might soon be the last occasion on which I would see her, but I never expected my healthier father to die first.

It is only natural that I would revisit the psychological landscape of the last night I saw him before his fall, again and again, because I believed that there must have been actions I might have taken to prevent my father's accident in the middle of the night. Logically, however, I was aware that I could not have brought back my mother from that other realm in which she was dwelling.

Chapter Five

Early Signs and Symptoms

Angry Gardener

Ripping up plants,
following diffuse root
systems until their caps
have been snapped off,
she breaks up soil, turning over clods,
stones thrown to one side, heaped in a pile
that clamors as another is sacrificed.
Dark landscape carpet is stamped flat,
subjugated by nails at corners,
before she casts down the course,
unconsolidated sediment
in clumps to be raked by jagged metal edges.
Heavy flagstone is dropped into place.
By now,
anger is diffused
in contemplation of arrangement,
obedient to the aesthetic
found in combinations of rock faces
scarred by age,
surviving fossils
of forgotten lives.

Gardeners have been compared to architects, caregivers, healers, artists, ambassadors, providers, nurturers, and as tribe; in fact, gardening seems to breed not only plants but metaphors related to beneficial practices of all kinds. Gardeners set out to help life grow, so it is only natural that we see work of the gardener in somewhat philosophical or even metaphysical terms. Human society as established is largely attributable to the work of the first gardeners who set out over the earth to cultivate and grow their food.

My mother used to love to work in her gardens. She knew the names of plants and flowers and tried to pass that information along, but I was resistant as a child. I just wasn't interested in botany or anything as seemingly passive as gardening. Years after Phyllis noted the names of flowering plants that I cannot recall, I wish I had paid attention to her when she was trying to impart her wisdom about gardening.

I can, however, revive the memories of my brothers wrestling and falling into her flower beds, matting down the plants, and then running for cover from her. At ten years old, I did not see the point of spending an afternoon in a flower garden, and I'm quite certain that neither did my younger brothers.

One of the qualities I remember about Mom's gardening is that it calmed her, usually made her more content, if only briefly. She had an artistic soul, a head and hands meant to create. Gardens are associated with beauty and order. Her life with her lively six children and all of her elementary school students must have been perceived as chaotic. Those scenes in her garden represented an occasion of harmony and peace and patterned placement.

I don't know exactly when she stopped gardening, but I do recollect looking at her miniature flower beds behind the house and seeing that the weeds had taken over, the flowers were brittle and dry, and her oasis was no more a place of beauty, but rather a little untended patch of disarray.

I did weed it halfheartedly for her now and then, but the action seemed to be such a losing battle with all of the other losses around us. The absurdity is that I recall thinking she did not appreciate my efforts. Now that thought seems ignoble. It is only after understanding more about her disease that I came to realize that she could not make those cause-and-effect connections that most of us take for granted. Her life was wildly flying in multiple directions, and I was still worried about being unappreciated.

Why didn't we ask her questions about why she was not planting flowers anymore? So many decisions made during that period seem clouded or strangled. I know if we asked a few questions, my father would jump to her defense, or she would appear upset with us for asking. She would respond that she was tired, that she had too much to do, and I looked askance at her, wondering how much she had to do in retirement. If I tried to approach my father when he was by himself in order to ask about the circumstances he was dealing with, he was deliberately evasive, or Mom would suddenly come up behind me with an angry look on her face. Her paranoia was pervasive.

I honestly believe that my father thought that she would recover from whatever was wrong with her, and they would, at some point, resume their lives together. He would take her to Florida again, make her happy, and get her out of the cold New York winters.

After Phyllis had been well settled into the assisted living facility, I took her for a walk around their outdoor garden. We followed a circular pattern, but it was a pretty path lined with a variety of plants and flowers. I asked Mom the name of a flower that she had once planted in her gardens, and she didn't respond. "You know this flower, Phyllis," I persisted. By then, I realized that it was easier for her if I called her by her name rather than "Mom," which appeared to confuse her.

At last, she just shrugged her shoulders and said, "I'm cold." I think the temperature was about eighty degrees that afternoon.

I'm not sure whether or not she was still able to name any of the plants she was once so familiar with or that the plants simply held no interest for her, but we passed by them again and again and they went unrecognized.

In the entrance to my parents' house, visitors were long greeted by a century-old rubber plant that my mother had rescued from my grandmother's house after the death of her parents. I never gave the resilient plant much notice until near the end of the era my mother had lived in her own house. Neglecting to water her plants, nearly all of them were in bad shape or already dead because I, too, would frequently forget to water them when I visited. That rubber plant, however, seemed immune to lack of proper care. It persisted against every slight and injury.

When I chose familiar items of Mom's to take to the assisted living facility to set up her room, I brought the rubber plant with me for her. During the three years my mother lived there, I remembered to water the plant, now and again overwatering it, as the telling leaves fell away and settled on the carpet. Later, when the head nurse at the assisted living facility told us that they could not continue to care for our mother at the facility because of her increasing physical needs, I took the old plant home with me because I could not take my mother, and my sister flew our mother to a nursing home out of state.

I don't do well with houseplants, managing to forget about them fairly quickly and find only incidentally that they have died. This rubber plant Centurion, however, thrived, growing a thicker stalk and taller, becoming so tall that it was problematic even having this plant in the house, but there was no possible way that I could let my mother's rubber plant die now. As of this writing, this plant stubbornly carries on, bending toward available light when someone remembers to open the blinds. My actions toward her plant would make my mother happy if she could know about this. In any event, I have taken to this resilient plant in a way that I have never cared for a plant before. Clearly the association of both my mother and grand-mother is tied up in this holdout from another era. Even as this old survivor sheds its shiny leaves and renews itself, it seems to encourage personification.

My mother as nurturer began to be unrecognizable, how-ever, as her dementia progressively altered her personality. Mom was fiercely proud of both her children and her grandchildren. She was always good to her grandchildren and children in gen-eral, and the relationship seemed to be sacred. When she began to sharply criticize her grandchildren and would grab one of them unexpectedly, we knew, rather than suspected, that she was not quite right. But we mistook Alzheimer's for the abruptness and impatience of "old age."

We continued to misinterpret those actions early on and allowed ourselves to be manipulated by Dad's explanations because he thought he was defending her by not acknowledg-ing the disease. We made one misjudgment after another: she was getting irritable and mean. Little did we understand that she was experiencing some of her early psychotic behaviors due slow brain-cell death.

Phyllis Marie's anger appeared more and more regularly with less and less provocation as her debilitation moved into a new stage. Again, I initially took in this knowledge, filtered as it was through the lens of a daughter who had no experience or knowledge of AD, dismissively at first, as another vestige of my mother growing old. I was not alone in suggesting with some disdain that she was getting too ill-tempered with kids because she was advancing in age. I was wrong.

If I could enter some fantastical time machine, I would go back and listen when my mother explained that her "purple azaleas growing on the bushes" behind our old house on Route 90 "are a kind of rhododendron." I hope I would pay more attention when she described the difference between the blue columbines and the bluebells. I'm not sure that I knew how to please her when I was young. I might have cut off a few stalks of gladiolus and brought them into our house to set in a vase on the kitchen table for her.

Chapter Six

You Look Like Your Mother

Association

All legs, long and lithe,
her tan torso gracefully soaring,
an eleven-year-old glides through
my backyard. A waiting woman
wraps her child in affection.

And like an echo,
I perceive my second child
dancing across a smiling stage,
disappearing in wings,
within a ponderous cloak.

Considering that stream
of reverberation,
I recall my first daughter
running in a field to catch
a softball in the sun. Further back,

All legs, I was at eleven
when I could outrun

my brothers, an invincible girl
rushing on a course of
expectation.

Echoes now whispers, going back,
as a photograph of my mother
in her Communion dress, with her hand
outstretched, one sylphlike foot
lifted off the ground in an aerial.

Fainter still, my grandmother's fugue:
her delicate pose in sepia tones
as she recedes from view,
an orphan windswept,
without antecedent.

In an old black-and-white photograph, enclosed in an Art Deco wooden tabletop, swing frame, Phyllis Marie is wearing a white, sleeveless dress with delicate black lace shaped like a fan opening across her breast. At her neck is a velvet black ribbon collar, accenting her fair skin and rich brown hair that curls softly at her bare shoulders.

Even without makeup—which she never wore, my mother at seventeen years old looked like a Hollywood ingenue. In the photograph, my father leans his handsome blonde head against hers; his right hand is wrapped around her small waist as if he would never let her go, and, of course, he never did. He had already been through the experience of war and was home with the girl of his dreams. His smile alone tells you that. Like the Mona Lisa's, however, her smile is harder to read. It always would be.

Years ago, when I was a child, my parents were going out to some event, and we had a babysitter come over. I could hear my mother coming down the stairs, even her step was altered by her high heels and lighter spirits. She was already wearing her sole, extravagant black wool coat with the fur collar, her cultured pearls circling her neck, her lips flushing red, and her dark hair pulled back to reveal such beauty. Looking up at her, I knew she was as glamorous as a movie star that night. Of course, that was only one night; more frequently, my mother moved in a light that was harsher and harder.

Rushing ahead in time, my mother sits with her back to me as I approach her in the nursing home. When the assisted living facility staff could no longer care for her needs, my mother was moved to a private nursing home near my younger sister in another state from her home. As a result of the distance between states, I had not seen her for some time, so I was surprised when I spotted the back of her head. I did not expect to see her pretty brown hair among all of the white-haired ladies in the common living room with her. From a distance, she looked too young to be there. Something was not right.

According to an article in the *Psychology and Mental Health Forum*, the risk of "developing Alzheimer's increases with age."[1] Early onset of the disease has been known to affect people in their forties and early fifties, however. Yet, the vast majority of those who get the disease are over sixty-five years of age, but it is not as if Alzheimer's is ever expected. Like the worst kind of thief, it moves in quietly, unnoticed, propping open a window and crawling into a room. I thought of how long we had lived with this disease without acknowledging it.

For years, I thought of my mother's beautiful, brown hair as a superpower. Few people would imagine or believe that she never colored it to hide gray. Both of my parents had always looked young for their ages, but my mother held onto that gift until nearly the end of her life. With the exception of the Alzheimer's, my mother's health was extremely good, even in the nursing home. Her blood pressure, her vitals, her hair and skin still radiating a degree of youth; she appeared much younger than her years. It struck me as such powerful irony. If, in fact, she had never gotten Alzheimer's, she had reason to expect to live for many more years in good health. The dreams she had of traveling with my father would have become their reality.

"You look just like your mother," the tall woman in a tan business suit said to me, but she directed her eyes toward my father. I was only five or six, but I remember the feeling of pride when people compared me to my beautiful mother. I also remember the twinge of regret, in that I wanted to "look like myself."

It was only years later—as a rebellious teen—that I began to really bristle at those compliments, comparing mother and daughter. I had stopped wanting to be compared to her and only sought to distinguish myself from her. By then, I was, like many teenagers, finding fault with my parents on a daily basis, making ready for the break that brings adulthood.

Yet I drew a portrait of us together during my teen years, the illustration bearing a striking resemblance. I was not a particularly good artist, but it was a particularly good likeness of both of us. When I look at that simple pencil drawing now, I am surprised by how much we looked alike. I am also mildly surprised by how similar were our career paths after I had worked so hard to distinguish and differentiate myself from her.

When my mother began to act strangely, we did not discern her illness but mistook her mood swings and sudden, strange actions as quirks of personality and advancing age. She had, for years, repeated stories from her life, so repetition was not indicative of any condition except the fact that we were about to revisit another event from her youth. Reading a line in Nabokov's autobiography, I smiled with recognition—the kind where you know the line could have been written by you: My mother, like Nabokov's, "cherished her own past with the same retrospective fervor that I now do her image."[2] Mom had most definitely cherished her past, and now it was all being lost to her.

Early signs of Alzheimer's might be noticed quickly by some, but my mother had long had a somewhat quirky even volatile personality. For as far back as I could capture the images distinctly, she experienced wide mood swings and sudden out-bursts, expressing hurt or anger with definitiveness. She could also be very loving and compassionate, kind and generous, but we were wary of her flashes of lightning.

Unintentionally, I gathered myself, pulling back, not want-ing to resemble my mother, particularly since her actions and words around the juncture of the death of my father were so uncomfortable, even abhorrent to me. Knowing that there is a genetic component to Alzheimer's—albeit one that is still not completely understood—I considered the burden of those genet-ics and wondered if I was looking at my own future as well as hers. This burden troubled many members of my family, and this knowledge of the genetic factor only increased the stress and tensions in dealing with the disease in our family.

Only after gaining some distance from interacting with my mother am I able to more accurately assess the gifts she gave to me. Some of those bounties were conscious, thought-ful, and deliberate; some were genetic or distributed as a result of witnessing life practices; and a few were earned through an inversion process I simply call stubborn resistance.

When I wake up early before the sun, before the chores of the day, with a ball of fire in my brain that impels me toward some creative endeavor, I recognize that will or drive or necessity is my mother's bequest.

But when I sense the fear rising as a result of the actual lightning bolt in the distance, and I manage to calm my own fears, that is my contribution, overcoming fears my mother gave me from her own apprehensions. She gave me much, much more, however. This lifelong love affair with words, with language, that is my mother's benefaction, but the voice I discovered in them does not resemble hers.

"You'll be wonderful with children," she said, telling me to become a teacher, and I resisted her guidance for years, driving down busy roads before turning back. And she was right, even though I did not want her to be when I was young.

Lists and organization: she is undoubtedly the reason that I have always arrived at appointments ahead of schedule, that I am prepared for the day and its events, and that I seldom forget significant dates or occasions.

Reacting against her unsentimental streak, however, I keep too much. My father's letter opener sits on my cluttered bookshelf. My older daughter's silver baby rattle looks out at me toward the surface of my writing desk. I don't recognize my mother in these features except through an understanding of my defiance.

Her politics seemed right to me even when I was a kid. Her sense of fairness and humanitarian conceptual scheme became mine even when she leaned in to listen to my father's more conservative voice. All of my siblings leaned more toward my mother's liberal politics than my father's, although we admittedly idolized him.

I acknowledge, however, that I spent most of my childhood and young adulthood fighting against her strong will and personality. My actions could be interpreted as efforts to break away from all her fierce individuality, occasionally—it seemed to me—presenting as vortex. Yet, I am forever grateful to my mother, and I might have told her when I was younger, if she had provided me that compass.

Chapter Seven

There's a Tornado in My Head

Tornado

There's a tornado
in my head.
Curiosity is lost.
Unintelligible lines float
beneath smooth surfaces,
turbulence and disconnection,
regardless of
heroic attempts to retrieve them,
the spirit refusing to give in,
but the mind unable
to reach back and deliver the goods.
As it is, the effort to correct effaces,
erasing all spontaneity and delight
in experience,
breathing ash
of existence.

Some part of me wants to hold back, protect myself from the ugliness that I unintentionally helped to create during this passage, but it would not be honest if I didn't go there. This scene started innocuously enough with a broken-down car and a request to borrow one of my parents' vehicles until mine was repaired. If I had known how broken I would feel later, I never would have asked to borrow that car.

Dad was still recovering from his stroke at the time, but he was home and making good progress under Mom's solicitous care. Phyllis Marie had suddenly and noticeably become more protective of her husband, which seemed logical since she had almost lost him. I never considered that asking to borrow their extra vehicle for a couple of days would be an additional strain on them, since dad could not yet drive because the sensation in his right foot had not fully returned. In other words, one of their cars was just sitting in their garage unused for weeks.

I was working at my computer when I looked out the window and saw my mom's white Lincoln pull up as if the car itself was angry. I was not surprised to see them because they often dropped in unexpectedly, but this felt unusual. When I opened the door for them, Mom pushed past me, and Dad appeared terribly upset, his head down, his eyes not meeting mine. Mom was pursing her pale lips together in anger.

"Where are the keys to your father's car?" she demanded, not saying hello.

"What?" I stupidly asked, her question not immediately registering.

"You're not stealing his car. He wants his car back now." She was moving around agitatedly, looking for something, I could only assume were keys.

There was no part of this insult that made any sense. For years, my dad had taken my four-wheel drive vehicle to his camp in Canada because he didn't want to wreck one of his new sedans on the rough roads he traveled in Quebec. My husband and I never even hesitated before giving him our two-week-old Explorer to take on his trip. There was a long-standing, unspoken agreement of helping family when anyone needed it, and my always generous father had offered his car to me on many occasions, even when I didn't need it. We would do the same.

Of course, I realized that something was wrong with my mother, but I wasn't looking for the right thing. My husband was even angrier than I was, as Phyllis Marie marched around our entry, demanding that I return the car right then. I told my teenage daughter to follow me down to my parents' house and pick me up after I delivered their car. My mother stormed out, and my father would not even look at me.

As I drove their car the few miles that separated our houses, I could feel my confusion fusing into anger that was gathering like threatening storm clouds. I was thinking about all the things I did for them, and this was how they were treating me. It was the kind of insult that felt like a slice out of my skin, and my face turned deep red, my heart pounding so hard that I had to stop at their garage door and gather myself for an instant before marching in and throwing their keys on the table between them.

"Here are the fucking keys to your car," I yelled, unable to stop. "You're unbelievable," I shouted to them. I never looked at my dad or noticed his slumping posture until it was too late. I also never talked to my parents that way or used that kind of language with them; it was like I didn't know who they were or who I was at that juncture.

In less time than my arm could shoot forward, my father went over, crumbling, landing hard on the floor. All of my anger dissipated and fear took its place. I was past scared that he was having a heart attack or another stroke, but as I reached for him, Mom slapped me. She kept slapping at me and screaming.

"Get away from him," she yelled hysterically. "You're killing him," she shouted as my own daughter entered her grandparents' house in disbelief.

"Mom, what's happened? What's wrong?" she said, almost pleading with me, as my mother continued to yell while I lifted Dad's head and offered him some water.

"You're killing him." As Emerson Sr. started to come around and sit up, I could feel my anger returning, but it was tempered by concern for my pale father and the shame that my daughter was witnessing this bizarre scene.

My mother continued to half scream, half cry out that I was killing my father. I sat with Dad for a few minutes and gave him more water. He was beginning to respond normally, but he said nothing for a few seconds. At last, he said that he was okay, shaking his head, tears in his eyes.

Once he responded and looked at me, I thought that he was going to be fine, and I could not stay there with Mom continuing to yell. I left them in their house and rode home with my daughter, who was quiet. I couldn't shake that feeling of near hatred for my mother that night. She had precipitated the incident. But there was another emotion at work, as well. I felt guilt. I knew that I was not simply a witness as my daughter had been, but that I had played a role in creating that awful scene. I reimagined the situation over and over, trapped in a reel stuck on rewind.

My parents drove up to my house the next day as if nothing had happened the day before, but I knew my father was aware that something was wrong with his wife. I even thought that maybe he had passed out because he felt guilt, too. He was so upset that he let Phyllis demand the car back for no reason, but he was too weak from his stroke to fight her.

I just misinterpreted what the problem was again. From the position of time and distance, I can see Phyllis's Alzheimer's raging, the disease that she had been fighting to mask until my father had his stroke. Then all of her energy went into trying to save him, and the disease's fury was released. It was not as if I couldn't tell that my mother was altered, but I believed it was psychological rather than biological.

The worst aspect of that terrible incident, however, was how I let my own feelings of hurt and betrayal coalesce into anger when my parents needed my help and understanding. The paranoia Mom exhibited in her fury I now recognize as classic symptoms of Alzheimer's, but at the time, I thought she was just being cruel and manipulative. I don't know if I was angrier with her because I lost my temper in front of my ailing father or in front of my daughter.

It was not a permanent break, however, and Mom still had days when she seemed to function relatively normally. They came over for dinner or boat rides on our little lake on many occasions after that incident, but something seemed like it snapped inside me. My feelings for my mother became increasingly testy and suspicious and angry. I regret that. She became increasingly paranoid. I regret that I didn't instantly forgive her and comfort her more. I wish I had pushed harder to get my father to take her to the doctors to get adequate medications.

When I did forgive her, she did not know it because she was too severely ill in the late stages of Alzheimer's. I sometimes recall the afternoon that felt like someone else's life not mine, like something out of a Eugene O'Neill tragedy. I think about how long Mom had to cover her symptoms, how frightened she must have been, and I want to cry. Dad's stroke took her remaining strength that she had been using to mask her disease.

I have to remind myself that I was a good daughter, a loving child to my parents, that there were plenty of instances when I reached out and assisted them. Logically, I know this, but I have tried so many times not to see that awful scene in my head. Still, it reappears on its own terms. If I could change nothing but my own actions, I would.

Chapter Eight

Helping the Doctor

In a Book's Spine

A book bent at its spine,
twisted backward,
tumbles out words
in a line:

"Amber
upset
didn't
convinced
named
stood
of William
who had
stolen
several
doubts
they told"

Looking
for a message in the randomness

of spilling, like Ursula LeGuin's
speaker searching for signification
in froth on the beach,
kicked up by ocean,
or meaning of intricate lines
found in a lace collar—
all these *Texts* we're
seeking to decipher
even when we know
answer is denied.

By the time we had convinced Dad to take Mom to a doctor to examine her, Phyllis Marie was diagnosed with mid-to-late-stage Alzheimer's disease. I began to realize just how remarkable my father was in caring for her at home all that time, without help, although he resisted our efforts to get help for him. When he finally worked up the resolve—and overcame his guilt—to take my mother to her physician for an Alzheimer's test, he was met with a system that is not intended for the secrecy, the deceptions unintentionally created by patients and their families who are dealing with this disease.

The honest appraisal and medical response to AD, in fact, made for hardships for Dad. Part of the problem lies with our legislation, as well, in which health care professionals cannot give out patient information to family members at all or only with a great deal of paperwork and official role designations and agitation expended.

When I tried to make an appointment for my mother to be tested for AD, I was rightly told that the doctor could not speak to me about my mother. Our legislation is in place to protect a patient's rights. Even though I understood this, I just wish the doctor could have spoken with me or my sister-in-law, rather than my mother, who refused to admit she had any problems. I honestly didn't know how we were ever going to get her into a doctor's office again once she became paranoid. It almost feels as if families experiencing Alzheimer's in their midst should have a legal exception, but then I am not sure how different the outcome would have been even if we were able to get her to the doctor's for diagnosis sooner. It might, however, have benefited my father, even saved his life.

I thought that it would be so helpful if my mother's medical practitioner could just have a casual conversation with Phyllis, evaluate her subtly, and then make out a prescription—state that it would help her health without explaining the fact that it was for her dementia, but then I have to consider the potential for abuse of patients' rights without these laws and protocols in place.

Unfortunately, this forthright evaluation was conducted during her most suspicious and aggressive stage of the disease. My mother always believed in the wisdom and sanctity of health care specialists, and she would have taken a medication gladly if she believed it aided her health before she got Alzheimer's. Instead, however, when the doctor revealed the fact that he was assessing her for dementia, she got very angry, insulting, and resistant.

She yelled, "I'm not crazy."

The doctor calmly asked one question after another, taking notes as he spoke and she stubbornly refused to answer. She became more defensive, although she was probably frightened that she could not remember very simple answers to routine questions.

Her coping mechanisms were in high gear, with her responses to questions such as, "Who is the current President of the U.S.," prompting her to state indignantly, "Well, of course I know. I'm not going to answer such ridiculous questions." She moved on without stating the name.

When the doctor finally asked her in what city she lived, my mother was unable to hide her confusion and seeming hostility. "I know where I live! Don't insult me," she shouted. Yet, she could not produce the name. It was a terrible moment when she looked at me with an accusatory, hateful eye. I recall trying to reassure her, smiling stupidly and helplessly, yes, feeling complicit with the doctor who was, after all, doing his job.

It must have been humiliating for her, however, even in a reduced capacity—to be asked such simple, almost juvenile questions and not be able to produce the answer. I later surmised that my mother's most hostile period—during the span in which she hit and yelled and threw things—was a fear reaction.

Sitting in the medical office with my father, I saw the effort it took for him to keep from falling apart in that matter of fact, clinical atmosphere which was devastating because of the nature of the information being presented. The doctor explained to him that there was no cure at that point in time, and that his wife would get progressively worse; he also suggested that Dad would need to find nursing home care for his wife. My father had managed to deceive others for so long that he must also have believed some of his own fabrications as to why Phyllis was acting the way she was.

I watched as Emerson Sr. cataloged what seemed to him were blows, moving from disbelief through sorrow to stubborn resolve not to cooperate with this man who would have him give his wife away. Any attempt on my part to agree with the reasonable doctor was discerned as collusion from Dad's point of view. Although mentally sound, he simply was not ready to listen to this diagnosis in this manner any more than she was.

Later, medications—which might have helped combat some of those behaviors associated with Alzheimer's—were prescribed, and my mother would not take them. She never willingly went to the doctor's again. This was a woman who had always taken her pills without question and held doctors in the highest regard. Suddenly, there was no subterfuge too great or a strategy that could trick her into taking her medication even in her confused state. She began emptying cups of tea before she drank them, checking her food for evidence of foreign, "poison" substances.

Following that visit, my mother became increasingly paranoid, whispering, secretive, and angrier. She began hiding possessions to a greater degree and writing strange notes. Part of the problem with treating patients with this ailment lies in the nature of the condition itself and part of our particular problem was how proud we were, initially unable to admit to my mother's failing health.

Typically, physicians are trained to deal honestly and openly with their patients, but Alzheimer's patients are sometimes intermittently paranoid at the onset of the condition. Although we should not have deceived ourselves, it would also seem that a little deception in dealing with the patient with Alzheimer's makes some practical sense in terms of management.

I learned eventually that the faster I talked to my mother, the more upset she became. The more I tried to reason with her, the more confused and angry she grew. The more I tried to help her locate, the more disorientation she manifested. On many occasions, both my father and I argued with her about her orientation, trying to convince her of where she lived and how old she was. I look back on those scenes with sadness. I wish I had just agreed with her and asked what we could do to make her feel more comfortable. What was important to Dad and me no longer held importance for her.

It makes sense to me now that if the totality of experience is jumbled for you, someone talking even faster about people and places you don't associate would be more disconcerting, even frightening.

I wish I could have asked my mother what she needed to eat or how warm she wanted to be rather than tell her that she was married and how many children and grandchildren she had. This reorientation came at a time when she saw herself as a child again, so telling her that she had grandchildren seemed impossible to her. Only much later did I begin to understand how terrifying it must have been for her during that stage when she was losing her connections with those individuals she had loved and that even the simplest of bodily functions—like picking up a fork to eat dinner or cleaning herself after eliminating—would no longer be possible without help.

When my father finally spoke to the doctor, with tears welling in his eyes—eyes that were fierce with protectiveness for my mother—he asked if there was anything, any medications that could help, that could reverse the process. Watching him try not to cry was agonizing for me because my father never cried; it was a point of honor for him.

The physician told my father the truth: that there were no medications that would reverse the damage, his wife was too far into the progression of the disease, that there was nothing he could do in terms of curing Phyllis, and that Emerson should start looking at alternative placements. "Of course," he said, "there are antipsychotics you can give her."

"She's not psychotic," said my father argumentatively and resolutely.

"Well, she will manifest those symptoms," the doctor said. And she did.

The most difficult thing was realizing that even with everything that was known about Alzheimer's, it wasn't enough to prevent the loss, the sadness, the slow, painful retreat from everyone and everything my mother had known.

Here is a statement of hopelessness: your wife, the mother of your children, as the woman you have known, is lost to you forever.

My father never accepted it.

At first, he guiltily tried to give her the antipsychotic drugs in her tea, but she always suspiciously looked at the tea then threw it out. It was as if she was convinced that he was trying to poison her. She began moving her food around on the plate and not tasting it. She hardly ate during that period, and I wondered how she remained as strong as she was, but her weight loss was rapid.

I assumed for a time that my father was giving my mother the drugs prescribed, but only much later found out about the dilemma he was having. He did not want to admit this either because he felt badly giving my mother drugs in the first place or because he didn't know how to do it in a way that was less threatening to her, less confrontation for both of them. My mother did not seem to respond to any of the medications because, quite simply, she was not getting them with any regularity or getting them at all.

Then Dad finally confessed that she was throwing out the medicine, and he inferred his betrayal to her. Emerson Sr. was right about one particular idea, however. Phyllis was throwing out her tea, and she believed her food and drinks were tainted. For as confused as she was, she remained surprisingly clever about watching what anyone was doing with her food or drink. Although I was able to "trick" her into drinking some of the tea with the medicine in it, she more often continued to push away what was offered to her.

Physicians certainly don't need medical advice from patients' families or laypersons outside their area of expertise, but perhaps they could benefit from reading about what the families as well as their patients with Alzheimer's experience.

What do I wish is to share this information with others who might go through this experience. It is the same list that I wish I could go back in time and give to my father and myself, as well as other people in close contact with my mother.

- Be kind and courteous—no matter how upset and stressed you feel—to the nurses and other health care professionals who will be caring for the Alzheimer's patient. That day-to-day contact is most difficult and requires tremendous patience and support from everyone involved.

- Treat the individual with Alzheimer's with all the respect and dignity you would if he or she was a CEO. (Dad was far better at this than me. It took me longer because I wasn't sure of her disease until after I spoke with the doctor.)

- Blunt the harshness of your statements by couching your terms. It only takes a few seconds more to think about how to present information. (I got progressively better at this, but was woefully inadequate when I first started dealing with my mother after the onset of her disease.)

- Talk openly and honestly to each other. Family members can provide a tremendous amount of information to one another and health care professionals if they remain honest and calm. (Of course, this is the tricky part—staying calm under the circumstances. By practicing, however, I got better at this, and so did my father.) By talking often with one another, family members can support each other rather than begin to feel isolated.

■ Do nothing suddenly to make the person with Alzheimer's more suspicious or agitated. It is possible to redirect a person with Alzheimer's. (It took me far too long to put this lesson into practice.)

■ Get all the information and sit down to plan out viable alternatives for people who are providing palliative care, even if the alternatives are only designed to make it easier for the caregiver. (I wish my father and I could have done this together. I think the simple task of making lists would have convinced him that he still had choices even if he did not like the alternatives.)

■ Direct caregivers to helpful literature or find sources of information on AD for caregivers and family members. Information empowers people, particularly when they feel so powerless and besieged by this disease.

■ Be gentle and compassionate to each other in discussing the disease's progress. Honesty is a virtue, particularly by the physician, but it is not the most important quality for everyone else involved in caregiving.

- Carefully explain to caregivers how to give medications to people with Alzheimer's disease. Caregivers and their supporting family members should make sure that everyone understands what the instructions are for giving the medications, particularly in the event that something happens to the primary caregiver, as was the case in our family. (We experienced a number of instances of confusion—too numerous to elaborate on here—when trying to administer my mother's medication.)

- Provide some suggestions for how the medication might be given to someone who is suspicious, since many people with AD manifest this trait.

- Family members should worry less about orienting the person with Alzheimer's and more about making the AD sufferer feel comfortable.

- Plan for extra time for everything related to dealing with the person who has Alzheimer's. (Even formerly simple tasks took many times longer after my mother had Alzheimer's and getting impatient with her only exacerbated the problem.)

- Family members need to recognize that simple tasks are no longer simple tasks for the person with Alzheimer's.

I would like to add that I have tremendous respect for the doctors, nurses, and aides who cared for my mother during her stay at both the assisted living facility and the nursing home. While tasked with extremely sensitive and difficult chores, they showed my mother kindness and managed her care to the degree that it was possible for them.

Chapter Nine

Icebergs in Paradise

Saint James Triad

One bare leg audaciously
draped over a cool metal frame,
a naked foot dangling, a sensuous
arm curled round a straight line,
women whose lives were utterly
unknowable, connections impossible,
without memory, each one had
her bronze eyes eternally cast
toward indifference and the
artificial world from which
their physical boundaries
were formed.

What is your earliest recollection? Not the crush you had on a first grader or your visit to your eccentric aunt's house in another state when you were six or seven. Go back further, deeper, until life experience gets thick and murky, tangled lines confusing events with strange colors and angles, the point where you don't quite have enough knowledge of the world to make conscious associations and retain them. These earliest memories remain fragmentary, like shards of glass unless an older family member walks in with an explanation, a timeline of the events.

You see a pair of brown shoes with tiny holes punched in the shiny leather. You can't extract why this detail comes to you, why it is the shoes and not the man until years later when your mother tells you that doctors used to make house calls, and this giant pediatrician came to your house to give you a shot: a massive needle that scared you, so you hid behind the heavy fabric drapery where your sight took in only the tips of his shoes as he tried to coax you. Finally, your mother tells you, she had to grab you and pull you out screaming from behind a curtain. So beneath the sights loosely cataloged by a three-year-old is a small trauma. Trauma informs memory.

Of course, as you age and mature, learn facts about the world and yourself, you become proficient at storing information and reflections, making complex associations that create meaning, refine meaning, and revise meaning. Early memories, however, have the look and feel of dreams, where things remain disjointed, appearing random and discomforting, even frightening. I have heard many people remark, "I wish I was a kid again," but I wonder to what age would they like to return? Very young children can be adventurous because they don't yet appreciate consequences, but they are also easily frightened.

Memory is so closely tied to identity that people who lose either their short- or long-term associations begin to question their sense of self. How we define ourselves is inextricably tied to our ability to restory events. Memory becomes our path to identity.

Our feelings tied to memory may cause great angst, sadness, and pain, too. A student of mine recently wrote a paper on her grandmother's memory loss. As she walked through the hospital doorway, she pushed, "the dingy pink curtain aside and entered the plague of memory."[1] Her line struck me at once and was so perfectly attuned to the emotions associated with the disease in which what we revive becomes the source of pain. It is through our mnemonic experiences that we travel in time, returning to places that make us feel both their acute absence, as well as horrific presence if the memory is abhorrent. The memory becomes a confrontation of a moment relived.

Yet memory is also suspect as representation of events, as stated in this quotation from *Wired Magazine*: "In the past decade, scientists have come to realize that our memories are not inert packets of data and they don't remain constant. Even though every memory feels like an honest representation, that sense of authenticity is the biggest lie of all."[2]

Of course, as philosophers, we could examine the concept of perception and what constitutes the real from the perceived reality, but the central thread is that we are who we are because we have memories—whether they are chemically induced or not.[3] Time may be a man-made construct that is entirely false and our discourse about it may be nothing more than language play, but we seem to need this architecture to navigate through life with some degree of sanity. Such philosophical puzzles, however, are of little use in dealing with someone who has lost her ideas about verb tense and self. We typically operate in our physical world with an acute sense of past and present, and this disappears for the person with Alzheimer's disease.

The neurons in my mother's brain were dying. Her short-circuited, short-term memory made it almost impossible for her to have a conversation, complete a simple task, recall relationships, or even read a statement before the words' representations vanished.

For years, Phyllis Marie's favorite hobby was completing crossword puzzles, and she was very good at finishing them. Her disease progressed slowly, and for a time, she could read the puzzle clues, but she could not retain the clue for a sufficient period in order to search for an answer. By the time she read the clue, the possible answers were forgotten. I remember trying to help her complete the crossword, and her increasing agitation with me. Then, she suddenly threw the book containing the puzzles on the floor. That once-pleasant challenge had become an unbearable loss.

A much more volatile situation occurred, however, when my mother was removed from her home environment. On our last trip to Canada, she became almost totally delusional. As my mother sat at the table with my father, brother, and me at three o'clock in the morning, she argued that she had been abandoned by her mother; she looked at me directly and asked why I had left her when she was only thirteen?

Although the three of us knew that Phyllis was having a psychotic episode, for her, the locale offered its own reality, and her daughter had become her dead mother, one who had betrayed her. The more my brother and I tried to tell her who she was and what our connections were, the more fiercely Phyllis fought against us. It was exhausting and terrifying. My father looked as if he would collapse from the weight of it. Only after I "gave up" and tried another tactic did it click for her. When I began to agree with her pronouncements, all of her fight and resolve disappeared, and she became quiet and passive. We were able to sleep even if only for a couple of hours.

Realizing over a lengthy term and distance, I wish we had not taken my mother out of her routines because those trips only further agitated and confused her mentation. Striking me much later—even the house she had loved and helped design was much too open and confusing for her at that point in her dementia.

When she wandered into the formal living room, she was no longer in her home but in a strange place. Walking outside, leaving a comfortable home or room for no apparent reason, is one of the manifestations that indicates the presence of Alzheimer's disease. Sometime after my mother's death, I read an account in the newspaper about a local woman who wandered out in the middle of the night and froze to death while her husband lay sleeping in their bed. I felt such empathy for the man and wished I could have told him: I understand, and you are not to blame.

Phyllis Marie's many unsuccessful endeavors to leave her house were the result of panic at nonrecognition of the once familiar. It is the most unsettling concept to realize that—for those with Alzheimer's—walking down the street toward some faraway destination was less intimidating, less terrifying in some ways, than standing without movement in a room in which there were no tangible links, and people and objects stood undefined as strangers in this strange land.

Because I could not get inside my mother's head, I could only imagine what caused her to react the way she did after contracting AD. She frequently appeared to be angry or intensely annoyed, suspicious of those whom she loved. In retrospect, I realize that what she was feeling was not anger as I know it, but terrifying angst, disorientation, and maddening confusion.

On the Other Side

Fear runs through a wall
Running water in a sink
the riddling flux
High-pitch of the hour
turning inward until
tick of a clock
becomes click of a tongue
on the roof of her mouth
Lips moving inside
a knotted veil
Ringing phone is
shock inhaled
Wind registers as
unidentified voice
Soul a hole in the
center of her palm

Chapter Ten

Managing at Home

Unpredictable

A lightning storm is a reminder—

the jagged flash expanding and collapsing,

a tree backlit in reverse shadow:
light dark, the eyes never adjusting
to flickering indecision.

After the electricity has gone out,
its angry competition—a fulmination hotter
at its origin than the surface of sun—
illuminates only a question.
The man-made kind suddenly
timorous in comparison—
electric charge breaking down air,
creating an unpredictable strike path.
Thunder rolling in like warfare

on the move until you're smack
in the thick of it, ducking. You exist,
paradoxically, in the midst of annihilation,

the whole world lit up, then disappearing

as if a madman toyed at the switch.

If I was gifted with knowledge of the future, I certainly would have made some changes in how I responded to my mother in her dementia. I wish that I had gone along with her delusional scenarios instead of trying to place her in chronology and remind her of the "realities" of her life. I realized much later during my mother's illness that our efforts to orient her only made her more frightened and paranoid. If this seems repetitive, it is restated because this remains the single factor I could have controlled and made a greater difference in how we all functioned in our family following the onset of my mother's dementia.

We should have agreed with her no matter how ridiculous her suggestion. I finally discovered that when I did not argue with her, she dropped the seeming conspiracies and intense agitation of paranoid behaviors. When I did concur with her statements, I found that she lapsed into silence and peculiar calm. For that moment, she did not have to fight, to struggle against overwhelming odds of disconnection.

My father insisted on keeping their lives as normal as possible for as long as he could reasonably do so, and even beyond that given allotment. He did not share his fears with us easily, and once, when we were in a boat on Lake Yser in Quebec, he turned off the motor and said in the quiet on that desolate morning, "Your mother is failing." He was silently crying, and

I could not think of a helpful comment of any kind, so I said, "I know." But he had to be in the middle of a lake, miles away from her, even to say those words out loud. Just to be able to admit that she was not herself—and never would be again—took tremendous courage on his part.

Dad's insistence that he take vacations with my mother became increasingly problematic. My youngest brother and I tried to get him to leave my mom with a home care worker when he went on his fishing trips, but he simply would not leave her, so Larry and I took them to their camp in Quebec. The trips were memorable for nearly all of the wrong reasons, as my mother's disease became increasingly more apparent and fraught with difficulties.

Why did my brother and I agree to a trip that we knew was tremendously hard, if not dangerous, for my parents? It sounds so simple now, but at the time, saying "no" was not an option. First, we loved our parents very much, and Dad had this command over us even when he was being most gentle. There was an implicit understanding that if he was asking, we would provide. Second, we kept thinking that this would be their last time at the camp Dad loved. At the time, I thought that Mom might die soon, and Dad wanted to go there with her for one last good-bye. I also think that part of me, like my father, unrealistically continued to believe that a different circumstance might cause the return of her memory, even if only temporarily.

The summer before, I actually turned down my father's second request to take him up to his camp. We had gone in July, and I said that he and Mom should stay home in August or go somewhere less perilous. Dad persuaded my aging aunt to take them, and I found out later that he had fallen, hit his head, knocked himself out, and that Phyllis had nearly fallen out of the boat and had almost killed them all by distracting them when they were driving. My aunt made the confessions later when she was out of her brother's hearing.

So that last summer of our father's life, my brother and I agreed to take them twice. When Larry and I were alone in the cabin with them, Dad could not hide Mom's strange actions and inappropriate words from us any longer. There were exhibitions of throwing items and hitting us with whatever was handy for no apparent reason, and the harder we tried to reason with her, the worse it got.

The trips—which were once sources of adventure and fun—became like suspended nightmares in which there were only scars to stitch and bruises to hide. We took turns staying in the cabin with Phyllis Marie and trying to keep her busy—which was becoming nearly impossible during that continuance of her most delusional state—while the other two people climbed into a little boat and fished on the silent, dark waters of that deep lake.

At the point when it was my turn for a break from care-giving, I walked out to the end of the dock and just took a deep breath. The air was crisp and sharp even in the middle of summer, with a purity that seemed to arise out of an earlier era in the history of Earth. I remember standing on that weath-ered gray dock and letting the relief wash over me as the wind chased away all of the black flies and other stinging, biting insects. There were whitecaps on the water now and a shift in the direction of the wind as the clouds swept across the horizon and the sky grew denser and darker.

Even with the approaching storm, it was so majestically beautiful that I could scarcely breathe. I nearly smiled for an instant when I suddenly heard the whoosh of wings above my head. An eagle swept right over me—that might have seemed like some symbolic offer of grace, but in its outstretched claws, the raptor held the remains of a rabbit. As I watched transfixed, the eagle lowered its head and tore the guts out of the animal, entrails streaming like ribbons in wind, falling into black water, before the giant bird disappeared with its prey into the forest. At that point, I identified with the rabbit. Of course, that is the natural world. It is often cruel and indifferent, and sometimes, I have felt more like the eagle.

There was an instant, however, on that last trip, that seemed to come out of a movie. Although Mom had not recognized Dad all week, he walked out to the last few boards of the dock with her. They sat in two chairs, side-by-side, looking out over calming water. As I quietly came up behind them to snap a photo, I saw that he reached out to hold her hand. Inexplicably, she didn't resist. Neither of them spoke; my dad held that extended pause in the lining of their lives where he must have said his good-byes.

■

Although most of the responsibility for my mother's care fell on my father, I shouldered some of the burden of changes in their lives, as well. Dad took my mother to my children's games, and I quickly climbed over other spectators to reach my rapidly disappearing mother. I was not sure if she knew where she was going. Typically I followed her and tried to subtly direct her toward a restroom. If I was too blatant, she would begin berating me loudly in public. It always made me cringe.

I remember the events that I missed in leaving to find her. A half-court shot my son made in a basketball game had to be described to me after I returned with Mom. When I followed her, I did so partly at my father's request, partly out of his concern for my mother's well-being, but I also followed her with growing resentment.

When she went into the restroom stall, she locked the door and couldn't get out on more than one occasion. I recall standing in the crowded school lavatory, trying to coax my mother into coming out, talking her through the procedure that would unlock the door while she became increasingly agitated, nearly hysterical because the door wouldn't open.

With the physical and emotional space to analyze my actions and responses now, I realize that my directions were simply a jumble of meaningless words to her. I worried about the girls standing around me, looking annoyed because they had to use the toilet, and my mother was causing turmoil, from my limited perspective. I considered how I was going to get under the stall door when, magically, it opened.

"You got out," I said, startled.

"Of course I got out," she said in disgust. "I know how to open a door." The length of the period she had struggled was absent from her thoughts as she left the crowded little room with her seeming dignity intact; her disgust with me evident, even as she had failed to wash her hands. I felt guilt at not making her wash them, but was grateful I hadn't had to crawl underneath the stall door to reach her.

I missed a lot of my son's highlights in sports because he was going through the peak of his athletic involvement in school during my mother's struggle with Alzheimer's, as it moved from an early-stage to full-blown end-stage disease. The battle I surmised was as much with my father, I realized later, as with my mother, because he was always compensating for her, refusing to admit the problem, at least not out loud because that would make the terrible change final, irrevocable.

Whenever Phyllis got up in a public place, Dad motioned for me to follow her. This repetitive action became one of the dominating memories during this period.

For years, Mom was angry that I was trailing her, and she would turn and accuse me, "You don't need to follow me like I'm a child!" Sometimes she would slap at me, flailing weakly.

"I'm not, Mom. I have to go to the restroom, too." She always sounded so logical and indignant initially that I was tempted to back off and leave her, but I did not. I knew that her course was erratic, at best. Infrequently, I had to direct her to the restroom as she wandered into another hallway. At moments, she had trouble with the door handle. The most difficult part was trying to help her without looking like I was helping her and drawing her ire.

There were incidents that, retrospectively, seem to have an almost comic feel, as in a theater of the absurd. On one of our last trips to Canada, I followed my mother into the public restroom. These trips were always fraught with problems in that I never knew exactly what was going to happen, even though there was some routine involved. I had gotten better at following her without it appearing that I was too close behind in order to forestall her increasing paranoia.

The excursion was going fine on this occasion until I looked down and saw all of my mother's clothes on the bathroom floor beneath the stall's door.

"Phyllis, do you need some help?" I asked.

She said, "No. I can't get the door open." I then had a picture of my mom walking out naked with all of the strangers standing there waiting to use the facilities. Abandoning my squeamishness, I managed to squirm under the door and up into the stall with her.

"Hi, Phyllis," I said, trying to sound nonchalant. "Let's put these back on."

Thankfully, she acquiesced on that occasion and allowed me to dress her. Trying to maneuver in that narrow space, straddled over the toilet, and wedging myself between my mother and the door, I maneuvered her shirt back on, pulled her pants up and tied the string. I stuffed her bra into my jacket pocket as I was struggling between laughing and crying. Thankfully, she had become quite passive as soon as I appeared in the stall with her.

People were staring at us when we emerged, but I realized that I had stopped worrying about their judgments. Letting go of my discomfort with what other people thought made it easier to care for her. As we climbed back in the car, Dad asked with concern—because we were gone for a considerable period—"Is everything Okay?"

Mom answered indignantly, "Of course. Why wouldn't it be?" It surprised me that her actions were so disconnected from her words during that period. She could say the most normal sounding remarks as she performed the oddest actions, or she would enact routine actions while saying the strangest remarks.

After numerous exertions, both physical and emotional, my father was persuaded by my sister-in-law and with some pressure from his children to hire a home health aide to care for my mother during the day while he was at work. Even that concession was hard fought as he inferred the action was somehow demeaning to his wife. Without someone there constantly to assist the person with Alzheimer's, dangerous actions are far more likely to take place.

At 6:00 a.m. during the middle of the week, my phone rang. It was an old high school friend who told me that he had just picked up my mother walking down the street in her nightgown about a mile from her home. He had taken her back to the house, but my father did not answer the door, so he called me. I hurried down to my parents' house and saw my dad looking very upset, because he had been sleeping so soundly that he had not heard her get up and leave.

Apparently, he woke to the noise of the phone, but by the time he got up, it had stopped ringing. I realized how exhausted he was by caring for my mother, and the fact that he had to be relentlessly vigilant when he was home with her—even in the middle of the night. When I told him about my friend bringing her home, he was even more distressed and could not believe that she had walked so far alone. "Oh, my Lord," he said almost inconsolable, but she was not injured and seemed indifferent to our concerns.

Fortunately, it was late spring and cool but not a cold morning. I put socks on her feet, which she let me do rather than slapping me away as she did with increasing frequency. As I was wrapping a blanket around her, Dad told me that she had done this before, but he had always woken up in time to get her before she got very far. He blamed himself for sleeping too heavily. The disease seemed to cast a cloak of blame and demand guilt from us all.

My sister-in-law suggested that we put latches on the doors to prevent Mom's escapes in the night. Then we realized that Dad might have difficulty getting the latches open quickly because he had suffered a stroke a couple of years before. His manual dexterity was still somewhat diminished, and I imagined the setting of a fire breaking out and neither of them able to open the doors. The idea of a strategically placed, inside door latch was abandoned.

Phyllis Marie managed—on too many occasions to count—to leave her house to go "home," as she said, heading out with increasing frequency. Recurrently she packed a suitcase; and with draining repetitiveness she just walked out.

I checked her suitcase once after Dad asked me to retrieve it from the garage, and I found an odd assortment of items. There was a shirt and a stapler, a pair of scissors and a toothbrush. I tried to envision how panicked my mother must have felt and how confused she was. Some aspects of her long-term memory remained as she repeatedly said she wanted to go to Binghamton, the city in which she had spent her childhood.

On a Saturday afternoon when I went over to have tea with her, she told me, "All the women are leaving Cortland." I asked her where they were going, and she said, "It's too cold, so all the women have left." I explained that women were living in Cortland—we had not moved at all, but that had no effect other than to further agitate her. Usually I would have given up trying to orient her, and the calm would descend on its own terms, seemingly disinterested in the situation.

During the period in which my dad knew—but could not identify—what was wrong with his wife, he could not bring himself to admit it, yet they occasionally traveled. Before I drove them to the airport on one eventful occasion, Dad asked me to check my mother's suitcase for appropriate clothes. He was worried that she would be embarrassed when she got to Florida and didn't have the right clothes to wear. I had to do this surreptitiously because she was very paranoid during this interval.

I would like to say that I knew what was causing her distress and that I was kind and patient with her, but this would not be accurate. I knew there was an imbalance, but I thought she was just getting old and strange, as if that was somehow a natural part of aging. In rifling through her suitcase, I found that she had no underwear and only a single pair of pants. She had nearly every pair of socks that she owned stuffed into the suitcase. I quickly repacked for her and drove them to the airport. When we got to the boarding line, a security guard asked my mother to step over to her. I went with her.

"What are these?" she asked, pulling out the longest and most menacing pair of metal knitting needles I had ever seen. "You can't take these on the plane."

"Those aren't mine. Someone must have put them in there," Mom said.

Amazingly, the security guard confiscated the sharp silver needles but let my parents board the plane. I still look back with awe on that TSA individual who showed both restraint and compassion. As I stood waving to my parents, I feared for their safe return. I knew the knitting needles were my mother's, but she had not knitted in over thirty years. They had been stored in the bottom of a cedar chest in her bedroom. Why had she reached deep into that chest and pulled them out? What processes were at work? It appeared as if she was trying desperately to reach into her own forgotten past to retrieve the tangled lines of that which was already lost.

A couple of years later, while talking with family members of other residents at the assisted living facility, I learned that so many of the families there had similar stories to tell about the odd item tucked away where it should not have been. One of the comforts I remember is hearing the other people talk about their experiences with their parents or family members who had Alzheimer's. Somehow, our common experiences made the journey feel less isolating for a time.

Alzheimer's is not gender specific in its manifestations. Men and women alike hide personal effects and pack suitcases filled with odd fragments of their lives, all traveling to some strange destination from which they will never return.

Demarcation

A straight line division—
blue above, black below—
like the boundary
of the horizon separating water and sky,
only black water
is deeper than the phantasm of clouds
moving in waves suggesting vastness
to leap into and start swimming,
but instead, you would drop
37,000 feet
before hitting
like an exploding
stone.
Wing pitch with a light at the tip—
insignificant—not enough
to light the way
but enough to suggest a pulse.
This demarcation between
land and sky—
only the other country
you think you see is vapor,
and the straight line is not straight at all
but curve of the earth,
and as for the sky, well,
it is a void she feels and can only imagine.

Chapter Eleven

What Would She Have Chosen?

Aura

Two suns touching as in an alien
world Venn diagram, the collision
resulting in the splash of reds, yellows,
oranges, the chromaticity more intense
than the heart of a forest fire that

sparks and leaps from sky into water
without quenching the value
of bloody reds rising over black-forested
hills, slowly submerging in living
lake, this duality contradicting everything

we know about our heliocentric universe,
but the eye takes in this
deceptive aura, this trick, we tell
ourselves, must signal one as imposter—
the yin, the anti-Christ, the dark materials

from strange air, present nevertheless
in that drowning sky as fire spreads

over our volatile horizon, not explained
as Betelgeuse supernova, a sun collapsing,
but as chimera of the limits of our sight.

After he had succumbed to the struggle from kidney failure that was set up by the pneumonia, which began with a punctured lung in an initially failed re-intubation procedure in the hospital after his fall, my father needed a suit to wear at his funeral. I slowly went through his closet to find the right blue suit, wondering which one my mother would have wanted him dressed in if she could have made that choice.

Always particular in her selections of apparel, she would have desired that he look his best even in death. During his later years, my father appeared rather dapper, but he had grown into that style after many years of my mother nagging him to change his clothes or buying the suits and shirts for him. Mom always knew that the color blue looked best on Dad, with his blond hair, and that he wore a hat particularly well, so she brought home wool fedoras, and she knew that a suede jacket in light brown better showed the color of his blue eyes. One of my last gifts to my father was a fedora, and I realized that he needed a new one because my mother had stopped buying them for him. Before the onset of Alzheimer's, Phyllis made sure that Emerson Sr. had socks that matched, that they held a thread of the color of his suits and ties, that his shirts were clean and well ironed.

In the area of ironing, I had some practice and uneven feelings. In the days before my parents could afford dry cleaning services, Phyllis Marie assigned me the task of ironing my father's shirts. I had to use spray starch, and Mom would come over to check the collars before I could hang up the shirts. Of course, she ironed, too, but there were so many chores in a family with six children, that ironing became routine for me. Eventually, I took some pride in my work and played imaginary games in which I timed myself to see how many shirts I could finish in an hour. While it may have been my chore, it was Mom who directed the cooking, cleaning, ironing, and general upkeep of our house, making sure that my father always had what he needed when he needed it.

All those years later, I found a pair of Dad's socks, but I realized that one was brown and the other blue, so I had to go searching for a missing sock. In sadness and frustration, I finally decided to buy him a new pair, even though no one would know it but me. I could only guess at my mother's indignation with me in making choices for her, for my father, the man she had loved and cared for over fifty years.

I recalled the many occasions during which my mother had sent my father back to his closet because she did not like the outfit he had chosen. He would smirk about it as if he mismatched his clothes just for the fun of it, just to test her reaction. A woman with fashion sense, my mother wanted her husband to show that style, even if he was far less concerned with it.

When my younger sister suggested that we take Mom to the funeral, it was a moment fraught with problems but absolutely necessary to my family that Phyllis Marie be present at the funeral of her husband. Phyllis Marie had just been moved to the assisted living facility, and I was terribly concerned that she might refuse to go back if we brought her to family surroundings. We knew she should be at her husband's funeral, and in some way, she was aware of death, but she insisted it was her uncle or her cousin who had died. I had the sense that she didn't quite get what all the fuss was about. She didn't seem very concerned, and it hurt.

Phyllis Marie spoke very little during the funeral and stood in line with her children as people passed by, offering their condolences. Nodding politely, she even allowed people to take her hands in theirs, and she appeared to be reacting normally, even cordially, but those closest to her knew that she was lost to the impact. Instead, of course, my mother appeared variously disinterested in the flurry of activity of mourning around her and nervously agitated about something she couldn't quite remember.

I don't believe that Phyllis Marie—with her memories firmly in place—could have endured the death of her husband Emerson. Just for a few moments in the funeral home, the disease served as a disguised blessing. She could not identify her husband's face in the death mask of the man who lay quietly in his coffin. For her, knowing or fully experiencing the volcano of loss was irrecoverable.

At last, Phyllis Marie said that she was tired, and my sister sat down with her before taking her back to the assisted living home. It was completely illogical of me to feel upset with my mother over her lack of responsiveness to my father's death, but that is also what I responded to that day. I both wanted to spare her the loss of the love of her life, and I wanted her to recognize and remember him. He deserved that, it seemed; yet, she did not deserve her aphasia or the loss of those she held dear.

Alzheimer's exhibits as disconnectedness and is therefore alienating. If my mother had been well at the time of my father's death, she would have been devastated, abandoning herself to inconsolable grief. I could only imagine what she would have done or said. My father was her world, the man she had forsaken all else for and devoted herself to for over fifty years.

Chapter Twelve

Did You See *The Notebook*?

When friends and colleagues learn that my mother has Alzheimer's, one of the first questions they tend to ask is, "Did you see *The Notebook*?"

They talk about James Garner's character quietly lying beside his wife who has remembered their love after he reads her passages from her notebook, and there is hardly a dry eye in the audience. They tell me about Gina Rowlands's role in the film that is directed by her son Nick Cassavetes, and her character Allie, who suddenly revives her love for her husband Noah before they die peacefully in each other's arms.

The problem with this film is that it does not accurately represent what happens with many people with dementia. The romanticized version allows the husband and wife to die peacefully in their sleep, beside each other. The reality is that the person with Alzheimer's or another form of dementia is most likely sleeping in separate quarters, and not even a notebook will bring back the memories that have disappeared due to atrophy of the cerebral cortex and gross amounts of amyloidal plaques and neurofibrillary tangles in the brain, and not an unwillingness to call personal history to mind. Still, I loved the film, too. It represented a wish or dream of what should be.

There was a stage in the progression of brain degeneration in my mother that was outright ugly. At first, I just thought my mother was getting mean in her advancing age, and her husband was so fatigued from the battle of fighting for recognition with an unknown enemy.

Dialogue from the film *The Notebook*,[1] according to a fan website, reveals the optimist's view of Alzheimer's.

She remembers, Doc.

I read to her
and she remembers.

Not always,
but she remembers.

But senile dementia
is irreversible.

It's degenerative.
After a certain point,
its victims don't come back.

Yeah, that's what
they keep telling me . . .

[Later in the film:]

I remember now.

It was us.

—It was us. It was us.

—*Oh, my darling.*

Oh my sweetheart.

I love you so much.

Oh, my baby.

Noah, Noah.

I love you, Angel.[2]

The miracle I wanted or wished for actually happens in this film, but not in life. Filmmakers have a right to portray fantasy, but I needed to distinguish between these realms and find ways of coping in the world outside the cinema.

Dialogue from a scene between a loving husband and wife follows:

> *You're an old man. Get out. Get away from me.*
> *I'm your husband. Don't you remember?*
> *I think I'd know if I was married, and I certainly*
> *   wouldn't marry an old man. Get out.*
> *I'm your husband.*
> *I don't know you. You're old. Why would I want an*
> *   old man?*

With so few laypersons actually understanding this affliction, clarity is important for family and friends who must deal with the realities of dementia on a day-to-day basis. A startling aspect of Alzheimer's is that it robs identity and the short-term associations before it takes away vocabulary. My mother could say the most cruel and intelligent-sounding statements, even though they were unrelated to the context of the conversation or contained the absolutely wrong emotional core. Sometimes, my father looked stricken by her words, and at other points, he was simply exasperated. Theirs was a love story, but the ending for them was neither gentle nor romantic.

Yet, I know why we return to the ideal that *The Notebook* and other fantasies offer. Such is the strength of the appeal, it is nearly impossible to work against it. I found in writing this book that I had to back up and begin again because of the need and desire to alter the ending, the intense longing to make order out of chaos, make meaning out of confusion, and attempt to fashion beauty out of ugliness and sadness. There was also the task of trying, without consciously directing it, to avoid blame where none existed. I have my father to thank for everything he did to protect my mother's dignity, but he was also largely responsible for the prolonged confusion that plagued each of us.

I believe that my father's love for my mother, in the face of all the exhausting, debilitating, irrational interactions between them after the onset of her suffering, demonstrates a kind of romanticism—the word that expresses the value of hope, emotion, and imagination over logic—that even the grandest films could not capture.

Lantern as Moon

Concealed by cryptic memory, a window
opens slowly with a lantern as moon
guiding my way down, down
steep banks to a black river
in icy cold of early spring,
our breaths frosty, our limbs excited
as we scampered over rocks leading
to water's edge; father holding out light

that caught silvered slivers flashing
in dark, our dip nets yawning
and anxious to scoop mouthfuls
of rainbow smelt into white pails,
catch of the luminous,
during this middle of the night run;
temperature plummeting, creek swollen;
my father and grandfather ventured out boldly
in hip-waders as my brothers and I leaned out
over rocks, peering into frenzy.
When our father reemerged,
holding a living net smelling of rivers
and powerful oils, my brothers slipped
their fingers into the bucket to mix
with wiggling fish. I plunged
both hands in, temptation so great
that I had forgotten
I was wearing my father's watch.
Pulling out, panicked,
I dried watch on my shirt,
ready to cry, but then
dove back into numbing cold.
Water alive.

On the banks along and above the bridge
were other fishermen, but night was still;
absoluteness of dark punctuated only
by narrow beams of lantern light,
insulating us
into humble communities,
 all hushed by experience and sudden bounty.
Mother waited at my grandparents'

green patchwork-shingled house
with a baby in her arms.
She never went on those nighttime
forgaing expeditions but was relieved
when we returned cold
and "talking a mile-a-minute."
Although my father cut
heads off little fishes,
spreading old newspapers over the table,
as we gathered around—recoiling at
these beheadings—it was my mother
who floured and fried fish.
I held my baby sister,
Grandma lopped off chunks of lard
to ladle into a cast iron skillet,
popping with the dance.
The beast of a ravenous stove, fed
with wood, heated kitchen until chill
became a distant relative.
I don't remember being hungry,
but we were excited
by the prospect of food.
I had no idea of the fears of adults
around me, only that they all seemed
part of the adventure.
We stayed up late, limits blown out,
and ate sweet, fresh fish, rare in days
when no one had money
but didn't know they were poor.

Until I woke one morning,
recognition of dream

a distant memory and memory
a dream of discovery
in which my father, mother,
brother, grandmother, and grandfather,
now long gone,
emerge vividly luminous
with us huddled together, first
concealed, then illuminated
by swings of a false moon.

Chapter Thirteen

What Not to Say

Composed on a Napkin

Composed on a napkin in a diner
after understanding arrived
too late to do anything except

reflect on scene: realizing only now—
the way Frank Conroy saw it years after he
witnessed shoeshine men staring off into
distance—that I should never have tried to
direct her, remind her that she was 72 not 36
and that she had been retired from teaching
for years, "No, Mom. You were not fired
yesterday. You weren't kicked out at all. See
this newspaper. What's the date?" I said as she
threw cookies (I'd just bought at the bakery)
at me, missing with three of them, only one
breaking against my forehead, Dad arriving home
to have her greet him, "Who are you? You're
an old man," when he remarked in that lost little
boy voice, "I'm your husband. Don't you
remember me?" Dad as bad as I was at getting this
right, not making the adjustment to having her

gone, the woman in the kitchen not even looking
like the one we knew, this woman's face
gaunt and pinched with strain in her brain,
deteriorating I-function that left her drowning
in a terrifying alien soup with no points of reference.
"No. I'm not your mother. I'm your daughter.
You have six grown children and eleven grandchildren,"
I said with an exasperation that must have been
experienced as a tornado rushing in at her,
only later finding her note, buried in the mess
of kitchen papers in a cupboard,
the hand-scratching I barely recognized, one
with a phone number for a suicide hotline—
all of it too late for anything except reflection
and invocation of a return to the past; a redo,
one in which I wrap my arms around her, tell my
dad that he looked dapper, then whisper to
my mother, "You look lovely today. Yes, you're 36.
Let's have a cup of tea with these cookies
that you made."

Any form of dementia is unlike other illnesses in that people often remain uncomfortable talking about it or offering sympathy to those affected by it. Even when well-meaning individuals want to help, they don't seem to know what to do. Unintentionally, they say hurtful things without realizing it. That was part of our lives for years.

An often heard comment that many people made on their first and typically last visit to see my mother in the assisted living facility was, "She recognized me. We had a nice conversation. Does she have to stay there? Why did you put her in here? It seems like she could live at home or with you, couldn't she?"

At first I was hurt and then angry. It felt like an accusation as I read the spoken and unspoken lines, "I see nothing wrong with your mother. Why did you commit her to a nursing home? Why don't you let her live with you? What kind of daughter are you, anyway?"

But I came to realize that people did not mean ill will; they just didn't know what to say, and they did not understand the disease. And it turns out that the conversation they had with her was not really fulfilling because they didn't visit her again. There are sign-in/sign-out sheets at the entrance desk for visitors, and I discovered again and again that I was the last person to visit my mother each week.

I have often wondered since that period of time what possesses people, what is that need to have someone recognize them, acknowledge their existence even when that other person is incapacitated?

What compels us to seek this kind of contact with others even when we don't follow through? Why is it so important for people to feel that they are recognized in this situation? I don't have any answers, just puzzling and troubling questions about human nature, our frailties and capacity for kindness and cruelty.

I came back to this question again and again, however: Why do people make the assumption—if it is incorrect—that she recognizes them? She does and she doesn't. There seems to be some face retention—because *recognition* is not quite the right word—for a lengthy period for people with this disease, but the context for that retention and the complex associations our brains make for us in weaving together our human relationships are tangled within the brain with Alzheimer's disease.

Alzheimer's alienates. Old friends stop coming over. The odd or unintentionally mean remark becomes breaking point, and it is relatively easy to stop visiting because it is so burden-some. It was hard to blame people for not visiting Phyllis Marie because I knew firsthand how difficult she was, how difficult the situation was.

My mother seemed to "know" me for a stretch during her illness, yet she seldom could identify me as her daughter or use my name. She simply stopped trying to come up with a name. On a few rare occasions, she used my name, but then she stated that I was her mother, not the other way around.

As early as three years before the time when I took her to an assisted living facility, my mother had said that I was her mother, and that I had abandoned her. Then she said she was an orphan. I was struck by the single thread of truth in the scenario she came up with on that miserable night when no one could sleep because she was so delusional. My grandmother had, according to my mother's early stories, been an orphan who was adopted.

But as my dad, and brother, and I tried to redirect her, she became increasingly upset, manifested as anger, finally accus-ing me of being her sister who never liked her, and accusing her husband of being a stranger, an old man. She said that she never married. That she was still a girl. On that night, all the threads of memory seemed to have been split and broken because my mother never had a sister, although she did have three daughters.

For many people with Alzheimer's and their caregivers and immediate family, the first stage feels like the beginning of dealing with grief: denial. We stayed in denial far too long. Eventually, we moved into anger and then crept gradually into depression. The only stage I never witnessed from either my mother, father, or those around her was acceptance of the disease during her lifetime. But unlike the loss associated with death, losing a sense of self, losing one's memory, is another type of loss, with an indefinite end.

For months after my father died, my mother never said his name or asked about him. To me, it appeared that he had never existed for her. Then, on a Sunday afternoon in her room at the assisted living facility, my mother suddenly blurted out, "Where's Emerson?" The dread rose up in me. How would I explain to her all that had happened? That her husband was dead? Would she question me about how he had fallen down the stairs? Would she remember that perhaps she had a role in his fatal fall? But just as I began trying to measure my words, she had moved on, forgotten the very question she had just posed. She did not say his name out loud to me again.

What was even more disconcerting is that she did not look upset when she asked about Emerson, but she stated it in the manner in which she had asked this question on a thousand other occasions in her life before the disease. Of course, she wanted to know where her husband was, but she could no longer remember who he was.

I recall looking for some point of intimacy in her eyes that I considered was there for an instant, but I don't know if that was wishful thinking on my part because in the next second, she had lost that solitary thread. I did not have to tell her about his death again. Her eyes were no longer shining, without inquiry. That hoped-for light had disappeared even before it could be identified. I composed myself and said, "He's not here." Dreading her next sentence, I tried to think of what I could say that would not devastate her, but she surprised me again.

"Who's not here?" she asked.

As long as I could keep up with her changes of direction without overtly positioning, our visits had finally become pleasant. Of course, she was now getting her proper medications, and she had stopped her bouts of sudden violence and abusive behaviors. After she began receiving the antipsychotic drugs that calm the terrible fears that must surface with the loss of connections, my mother became gentle, almost sweet.

Over time, she spoke less and less frequently until, finally—years later, she seldom spoke at all. She could "rally" to try to look at you when you came to visit, but you knew that she was pulling out of a deep, thick fog. There were no more arguments, no yelling, nor crying, no negotiating. Even if she was able to say anything, I could not detect my mother in the spoken words. Her battle was lost.

The problem was that this passive woman did not resemble my mother in character or personality. My mother would have demanded answers, complained about her care, questioned what was going on, asked everyone, and sorrowed deeply and immeasurably over her husband's death. Emerson was lost to her in a way that even death could not penetrate.

A sole consolation I allowed myself throughout that terrible period was that my mother was spared the mourning she would have gone through if she had realized that her husband had died in a fall down to their basement. She was spared the cruel knowledge that she had left him there on the cold cement floor and walked down their street to nowhere. She would never again be cognizant that she was wandering about town in her nightgown, and that she had, quite possibly, played a part in the death of the man she had deeply loved.

I thought of these things as I sat there with her. It is taxing to visit a person with Alzheimer's because you can't feel them make connections either. I had to look for intrinsic rewards, knowing that I was somehow a comfort and that my contact made my mother feel less lonely if such a condition could even be quantified or qualified for her. I do believe that people with AD feel a kinship with loneliness, even if they can't categorize it or correctly identify it. She seemed more at peace when I was there after I learned how to read her gestures.

What should a family friend say to you after visiting your mother in a nursing home? Simply that she came and spoke to your mother, that she cared, and that she will come back to see her again next Thursday—or whatever day works. A few of her friends sent letters that I read to Phyllis Marie. It gave us diversions—labors to share, and I always appreciated those individuals for writing to her.

What counts the most is the presence, however, and what hurts—and is to be avoided—is to be judged. And, no, as a family friend you do not know more about the person's condition than the members of the family who have been living with this nightmare that is weighed with such portent, grief, and tension for such an extended time. The occasional appropriate response—out of conditioning—does not constitute a return to mental acuity.

Visiting an elderly woman whom I have known since childhood, I was taken aback when this typically kind lady remarked suddenly, "We had to kick your mother out of our bridge club. She forgot all the cards, and no one wanted to be her partner. It was just impossible to complete the game with her. She wasn't very happy about it, I'm afraid."

Initially, I was stunned and remained silent. Of course my mother would have lost track of the suit she was playing and all the other intricacies of a game like bridge, and it was a given that she would have to leave those pleasant evenings with friends behind, but why state the obvious?

"She was ruining our games, our whole evening, really," she added for emphasis. "She kept interrupting people, too."

"Yes," I said, thinking about all of those lovely women sitting around and criticizing my mother's errors and faux pas. "It's hard to decide what card to play when your memories have been robbed," I said.

"Well, perhaps she should have quit earlier." There it was. My mother and her family were to blame for the awkwardness of the situation—this terrible social lapse in etiquette of knowing the exact moment when to bow out gracefully and swiftly. Yet, there is no grace in Alzheimer's, I wanted to tell this woman but did not. They had been friends.

Since that evening when I said not a word to defend either my mother or my family, I have thought of responses I wish I had said, in reflection, such as, "How fortunate for you that you were not the person to contract this disease, and you were not the person whose connections to history, place, identity, and people were increasingly fragmented and short-circuited, disappearing, leaving you a living ghost. How fortunate for you that it was someone else and not you the group was gossiping about and ostracizing." I recall driving home and imagining all these insults I could have hurled at this former friend of my mother's, and now I am glad that I did not say anything.

Of course, I don't really wish I had said those hurtful statements because I had always liked the woman, yet I wished I could have shown her how distressing that condemnation and brutal rejection was for my mother and her family. My mother had never said a word about the bridge group again, even early in her trials when she was still aware of those slights.

Feeling protective of my mother when I considered those daily assaults on her dignity in the days when she could comprehend them as insults, even if she was confused about the circumstances, I am wide-eyed cognizant that I offered her no protection at all.

Merciful

Crow clawing at the door, wood-burning stove: a violation
This blackened black bird scratching at intervals.
Waiting for something or someone
to break into dark, facilitate escape, crow's torment
also tormenting: this mean talisman unwrapping its soot-soaked
wings like a drowning moth, worse than that fly—
Dickinson's disquiet, worse yet for its accidental nature.

Unlike this trapped bird, scratching out gore,
we can open the door, let the bird fly right at us,
measure odor of old charring,
wrap a cloth around the opening,
capture irrational panic before releasing tension into air,
although crow's thickened shape lays on the steps.
At last, merciful.

Chapter Fourteen

Managing in a Nursing Home or Assisted Living Facility

Cognito Ergo Sum

I try to imagine
my mother behind those opaque eyes
separating us from diseased brain.

"Hi, Mom."
"Don't tell me!"
We could be in separate rooms having
disassociated conversations,
so great is the disconnect.
I am continually at a loss at her side.
She seems to enjoy good food, however,
taking up the cheese sandwich until
reaching the point where the brain
loses track of goal, the sandwich suspended
until I guide her hand to her open mouth,
and I recall the sight of a bird feeding its chick.

I engage in the experience of moving
in and out of this signification of my mother

and her shadowy doppelgänger.
"I don't have a daughter.
I'm not married! I'm only 13!"
Then 79 then 13 then 7,
and I am along for this tormented journey:
an image of a girl in a country kitchen
at cheap Formica table shelling peas.
Her mother scoops up the work
of daughter, rinsing peas
grown in their garden—as real
as the pungency of urine
with the old man, strapped to his chair,
nodding his white head near us;
sensations of her reading to me as
I am reading to her—child's greatest fears
of abandonment.

This ritual at the end
knows no boundaries of time or place.
I think: patience, the powerful
elicitor of love.

On the first few occasions when I visited Mom in the assisted living facility, I was nervous because I kept expecting her to ask to go home. I planned what I would say if she asked, but it amazed me that she never brought up that subject. Early on, I took Mom on short trips away from the facility and found that she was never averse to returning.

She indicated through her body language and gestures that she was more comfortable in the assisted living home than she had been in her own house. It also surprised me that she had become so much easier to be around, simply because she was now getting her medications on a regular schedule—a routine that had been too hard for my father to manage. Once her routine was set, her needs met, her medications properly administered, she seemed more peaceful.

When I began visiting my mother multiple times a week, I had to come up with things to do that made it possible for me because it was hard. Some days I read to her, some days I talked about events, but they never engaged her on any level. When I discovered the diversion of excursions, I started taking her on short trips that she seemed to enjoy. I came up with a list of places we could go without presenting too many problems.

The only real difficulty in taking her on these little trips to ice cream shops and other stores was getting her in and out of my vehicle because it was an SUV that sits higher than a sedan. When I told her that I was going to pick her up and lift her into the vehicle, she allowed me to do that without fighting me. That action could never have happened just a few months earlier, but her disease was progressing, and she was becoming more passive. In addition, she had lost a lot of weight.

A trip to the ice cream shop seemed to be a favorite, and it provided one of the few occasions when she would actually state that she liked what we were doing. "This is delicious," she would say, eating her cone. She was losing weight so rapidly during this period because her interest in food had dropped off significantly, so any time I could coax her into consuming more calories was a positive.

Other trips that were very successful included driving by the Waterworks Park, where you could see the deer inside the fence. I'm not sure she saw the deer, but when I asked if she noticed them, she always responded, "Yes." On sunny days, I just drove her around through the countryside, and she seemed to like to look out, provided the windows were all up and the wind was not blowing on her. It was hard for me to get used to the very warm temperature she now preferred. She never complained that it was hot, only that she was chilled.

Within the facility, I took her on walking trips down other hallways outside of the Alzheimer's unit where we looked at the paintings on the wall. Most of the paintings—and there were many of them—were of innocuous, natural subjects, trees and streams, girls picking flowers. I had by then discovered that I could be slightly dishonest in order to amuse her, and I told Mom that we were in an art gallery. As I gently held her arm for her balance, we walked around surveying the colors and subjects. At one point, however, her old personality seemed to surface when she said loudly, "Well, this isn't much of an art gallery, is it?" I started to laugh, but my laughter startled her, so I refrained.

In addition to trying to engage and amuse her, I felt a responsibility for her physical appearance. Initially, this seemed foreign to me. I had to get used to checking on Mom's clothing, hair, teeth, and helping her with basic care. The facility's staff members were all very kind and responsible people, but they were burdened with many responsibilities. I learned to make sure that her hair was nicely brushed. Sometimes she was soiled when I came into her room. The attention I gave her regarding intimate personal hygiene, however, felt like the most powerful gesture of returning love. Through these actions, all of the old hurts passed, the tendrils of love returned.

I realized that in the process of caring for her in this very direct way, I was actually forgiving her and myself for our struggles during her combative period. Gradually, I took pride in making sure things were done well for her. After learning the hard way, I set up and paid for appointments with a beautician to do my mother's hair on a regular basis.

This was a task that I had not considered until a Wednesday evening when I arrived in Mom's room and found her pretty brown hair all chopped off, her bangs cut straight across like a little boy's. She couldn't tell them, I realized, how she wanted her cut. I set up regular hair appointments for her and detailed how to style her hair. I knew then that I was not angry with the woman who cut her hair but the situation that led to such results.

My dad had always maintained that, "people are basically good," but my experiences caused me to be a bit more cynical. It doesn't take too much analysis, however, to remember that the nurses, aides, and other health care professionals are human beings who react to stress and irrational demands just like everyone else. And they react to small kindnesses and appreciation, as well.

As a result of these observations, I made it a point to get to know the staff members by name, ask about their interests, and develop friendly relationships with them. I got to know Mom's nurses and aides, as they were getting to know what my mother used to be like. The nurses and aides always told me that Phyllis Marie was a favorite. I gradually realized that I needed to be my mother's voice and advocate because I knew that their job, too, was incredibly difficult.

After Mom had lost the power of her reasoning and ability to carry on a conversation, after aphasia set in, she could still sing with such power and beauty, extracting the words to songs from her childhood and young adulthood. It was initially shocking to her hear her sing these songs. As I listened to the other people in the facility, I realized that nearly all of them could repeat the words to songs when they could not recall the names of the children in their families. I discovered that the ability to sing originates in another part of the brain from our speech creation.

It was very unsettling, however, to listen to Mom sing the words to "Moon River," but not know who I was or that her husband had died. In one of the many odd coincidences of life, one of her favorite singers—Andy Williams—died in the same year as my mother. I thought about his only later, but look back now in reflection. Listening to her sing, it struck me that she was unable to know where she was, who I was, or be aware that her beloved husband had died, yet her voice was clear and strong.

Sitting with my mother in the common room at the assisted living home, I was delighted to see a sweet little girl take out her violin and begin playing for the residents. My mother and I had just sipped our tea together, and for a few moments, it became a familiar, even comforting, tableau, except for the strangers around us. The child was only about nine or ten years old and played very well, the high voice of the violin tugging at your heart.

My mother's face looked serene, and I adjusted the pillows under her arms in the chair (because she bruised easily), when she suddenly and loudly blurted out, "That noise is terrible. Who told her she could play?" I was so shocked that I didn't react immediately.

The girl stopped, and then looked at her mother and me. Her mother turned her away from us, but I tried to smile at the child, feeling guilt over that which I could not control. Mom did not stop, however, as she said, "What's she making that awful racket for? She's terrible." I knew from previous incidences with Mom that trying to quiet her would only make her response louder. I had discovered almost by accident that ignoring her remarks were the best way to contain them.

"Please keep playing," I asked the child. "She doesn't mean it. I know that she would love to hear you just as much as the rest of us, but she doesn't really know what she is saying right now." Although my mother certainly sounded rational and as if she meant it, I knew that she would never have made such a cruel remark without the changes in her brain. She loved children and music.

"Stop that awful sound," Phyllis spoke, even after the girl had stopped playing. Agonizing seconds that were perceived as minutes, and the girl walked over to another part of the room. I apologized to her mother and the little girl, but the woman shook her head and then frowned at me. I was so frustrated and upset by the fact that the more I wanted to quiet my mom, the louder she yelled and heaped abuse on the little girl. I had not yet learned how to quickly distract her. It was as if her brain needed a new route to follow, and I provided no paths.

The oddity of the display was all the more acute because my mother had been an elementary school teacher who loved her students. She would never want to say anything hurtful to any of them. But it wasn't simply about a lack of filters caused by the pathosis. The little girl playing the violin knew her instrument and played it well. There were no squawks or missed notes that are typical with children who are learning to play the violin.

Only later did I question: What was my mother hearing? Her strident criticism seemed to have no relationship to the child's playing at all, and I recognized another facet of this disease. The person with Alzheimer's may be sitting in the same room with you and appear to be listening to the same sounds, but their "thoughts" are located somewhere else, and what they hear is in another location. What they respond to is another type of stimuli entirely.

I'd like to write that my mother's remarks had no ill effects, but it was the last time I heard that child play for the group in the common room. I hope she came back on another day. That experience made me think about another loss. My mother hurt others, and they would be unaware that it was not really her making those seemingly mean comments.

During the severest period of my mother's illness, my father's youngest brother died of cancer, my cousin died—perhaps murdered—although it was never determined, my father died after a terrible fall, my father's youngest sister died of pneumonia, and, my dear younger brother died. There were times, during low points in this devastating period, when I would look quietly at my mother sitting in a chair with her distant gaze and wonder if Alzheimer's could be a relief. Of course, I knew that was not true, it only provided another level of dysphoria.

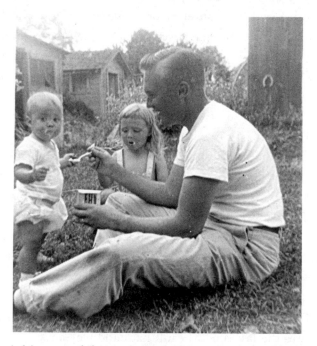

Figure 4. My young father is shown feeding me and my older sister ice cream when I was one year old.

Anecdotes to Loss

Disembodied voices calling
for passengers to board—
Istanbul, Cuenca, Ecuador—
but I'm waiting
for Detroit Metro Wayne County.

I purchase Moira Kalman's Principles of Uncertainty,
read, "My husband died at the age of 49.
I could have collapsed thinking about that."
I close her pages.

"Yes, yes, the tree-boring cerambycid.
You need to take the beetles out of the freezer."
He gestures talking to an assistant
in a faraway city. I imagine the other man
spilling insects across the lab's floor.

Here a Vietnamese family sits down, clutching
their bags, speaking words I can't decipher—
only their agitated tone.

A man to my right, talking in Arabic;
he is shouting, pushes away
from his seat, taking off.

To the left, a French couple—perhaps from Quebec?
Their syllables roll gently
as endings hover and disappear.

Deborah Digges's line in my head:
"And so it goes, like conversations in an airport in a dream."

A sparrow darts down from the tangle
of pipes and tubes above and examines this other world
as if it was city park and not a terminal.
The tiny bird pecks at a sunflower seed
spit out by a muttering teen.

A 4-year-old crawls under the table
where I sit, catching a word that wriggles.
When she looks up, she stops,
stares, wide dark eyes smile.
Her families' eyes, directed my way,
anticipate, interpret reaction—
sighs of relief all around.
Distracted again, they retreat
to their private sphere.
I am already imagining the child's life somewhere
far away, her family flown here by what imperative?

I scan rolling lines of arrivals
and departures;
time between
planes like purgatory.

A deck of cards flutters
in fluid hands of an expert.
In shades and a cool hat, he calls out,
"All spades,"
laying them down.

A cockroach manages
to avoid a thousand feet—

stopping, scurrying,
stopping, crawling until
it reaches the lip of a counter,
its miraculous escape, once again.

What would it be like to wake
like Gregor Samsa and find yourself an insect?
Stopping and starting,
scurrying for planes—
last call.

I take the next moving walkway
to my fate, I mean, my gate—
what a Freudian slip!
There is the STAND side and WALK side.
I have this perverse
notion to walk against the stand command.

At the end of a movable transport,
there is a bar
with ridiculous élan—
wooden veneers that appear
carved from another era.

Transparency walking,
night falling,
light shifting restlessly.

On the wall a billboard of Gwyneth Paltrow
dressed in white, holding white Labrador pups,
softness to the photograph—airbrushed.

In black letters, the advertisement's message:
I live for moments like this.

Opening Kalman's book again,
I lose my separateness in her variously wonderful
and grotesque drawings—
this one of a wide nun in black
on a bright yellow background.
How does she know
this juxtaposition will make us laugh
and mourn?

A line descends,
appears out of nowhere;
another plane lands;
a notebook flies open,
pages fluttering.

Deborah Digges flew once
from the top of bleachers.
I didn't see her descent,
only knew her aerials.

I'm well into Kalman's read
when I bookmark a passage with my boarding pass:
How are we all so brave
as to take step after step? . . . Bravery is suicide
on one end of the spectrum of existence,
and bravery is endurance at the other.[1]

It's boarding time.
Waiting for takeoff,

I open to the back of another book—
a note on the typeface—cursorial—
something about elegance, movement.

Chapter Fifteen

Collecting Memories

Before I Knew My Father . . .

Before I knew my father,
He was a bare-chested boy who could fish
by sliding his hand up underneath
an embankment and the fat,
white belly of a nesting trout.

He was a farm boy who walked 5 miles
uphill, but not barefoot, as he sometimes said,
during the glistening Upstate winters,
just to be the smallest guard
on a basketball team.

He was a young hunter who had tracked
buck for miles above the ridges
between Maine and Newark Valley,
when he surprised a doe nibbling on grass,
only to lower his rifle.

He was a 17-year-old boy who
knew nothing but courage
as he entered the Great War to find

justice for his big brother who'd already
lost his life on the shores of Saipan.

He was a blond-haired, angel-faced boy
who sat in the belly of an airplane listening
for shuddering flak on metal skin.
He was a boy returned from unrecognizable
contours of a newly shaped world.

He was a sunburned and willowy boy
who was dreaming of my mother when he
woke to write to her of the murmur
in his heart caused not by defect
but by love.

James Garner's Noah had nothing on my father as a romantic husband, even when my mother was unable to recognize him. The night before Dad died, I was at their house, standing in their kitchen, as my father told my mother that he loved her and undertook the monumental task of connecting with her, trying to help her remember their years together. He persisted, when many would have turned away in disgust or frustration. It seemed, in fact, that he would never give up, believing that she would come back to him.

When Mom seemed to stubbornly refuse to acknowledge his remarks, what he said was so filled with longing, sadness, and forgiveness of her inadvertent cruelty that it broke my heart.

Yet, I had no idea what a romantic he had been until after his death when I found the letter he had written to my mother when they were young. It was neatly folded in a box on a shelf in the closet. I had been looking for important papers after my father's death, trying to make sure that I didn't miss a document Phyllis Marie would need for her care. I also wanted to find some items to set out at Emerson Sr.'s funeral. But the letter was unexpected. I knew my parents well but knew very little of the interiority of their love. My mother had saved an entire box of his old letters.

After serving in World War II, Emerson Roy Avery was leaving the service to return home, and he wrote to my mother that he was sick with a fever. The letter stated that she needn't worry, however, because his illness was not caused by any sickness the doctor recognized or could cure. He wrote the lines that the murmur in his heart was not irregular due to illness, but out of love for her. I sat down in my father's closet and balled uncontrollably that afternoon. Yet, I also knew that this discovery of the letter was a gift. On that terribly sad day, I had found a source of their joy.

Because of my mother's illness, she was, of course, unable to make any decisions as to how to deal with their house, my father's estate, his law practice which had to be closed, their possessions, and her care. My siblings all came home from out of town or out of state to help, but it was as if some part of each of us was paralyzed from making the kind of smart and rational decisions we normally made as a matter-of-course. The compounded grief of losing both our parents at the same time just set us further apart instead of bringing us closer.

I thought about what happens to many marriages when a child dies. The likelihood of the marriage surviving such sadness is terribly diminished. One study suggests that the rate of divorce after the loss of a child is as high as 80 percent to 90 percent.[1] Grief has this way of driving wedges between people who otherwise love and care for each other.

My youngest brother and I drove my mother to her new home in the assisted living facility after first setting up her favorite furniture to look as much like a room in her old house as we could create. As we were driving, my normally talkative mother sat very quietly. I was actually frightened of what she might say, and I could hear my father's voice in my head, a voice that suggested I was betraying them both. It was one of the most agonizing short drives of my life, in which silence hung like trapped, angry wasps.

Although we anticipated my mother's anger or hurt, she expressed neither when we got to the Alzheimer's unit of the facility. She did not comment on the room's size, her furniture waiting for her, or the other people. After we had lunch together, I said that I had to leave, and she said rather matter-of-factly, "Well, leave then." She didn't watch me go, never turned her head in my direction, and did not cry out. The sense of betrayal I felt was palpable. Even though I knew that my mother's needs were being met, that she was warm and clean, that she was well fed and provided with good health care, that she was visited by me and a few others, I lived with guilt that settled into the space between my shoulder blades for the next several years.

A friend of mine at work recently told me about a blood test that she had, revealing some disturbing results. It appears that her liver is not functioning as well as it should be. The day she got the news from the doctor's office was the same day that she was scheduled to have a FaceTime interview for a new job. "I can't believe I have to deal with this right now," she said. "It's like my body is betraying me." Her words haunted.

Considering her remark, I thought about how all of us feel when our bodies appear to betray us. We develop blood clots that move to our lungs or our hearts. We come down with illnesses that set up pneumonia. Our bones break spontaneously as we age. Our bodies fail us, but it's not personal.

I also assumed that my father—even in what seemed to me at the time misguided intent—never betrayed my mother.

Such dedication required from him a kind of courage—as well as physical demand—that is difficult to locate. I only wish that my mother could have seen this courage in him, appreciated the kind of choices he was making for her. I only wish that she had never gotten Alzheimer's.

The disease, however, allows little if any closure—a word given far too much weight and repetition in our culture but, nevertheless, apt when it comes to describing the need we have to find an ending if not relief. With Alzheimer's, death is the only ending—although that may be said of all of us, in the final analysis.

Writer Margaret Atwood wrote an ironic short story titled "Happy Endings," in which she makes the claim: "The only authentic ending is the one provided here: *John and Mary die. John and Mary die. John and Mary die.*"[2] We all end up at the same point, but we rationally or irrationally resist, fight at altering that ending in some meaningful way.

Sorting through my dad's office after his death, I came across some of his favorite maps. I was supposed to be looking for tax papers and other papers related to my mother's inheritance. I kept getting sidetracked, however. It was strange how certain items, in particular, would cause the bottom to drop out.

During his lifetime, I was only vaguely aware of his love of maps. I knew there was a wall-sized, antique map of Cortland County up in his office at work. I was aware of his maps of Canada, which were framed in his office at home, but I never really thought about what those maps meant to him, never asked him about them. In looking through his papers, however, I found antique maps, maps of places he had been, maps of the counties in which he practiced law, maps that indicated the best restaurants, maps that located where trout lay in the deepest waters in his favorite lakes in Quebec.

All the Features of Heaven and Earth

Tracing the gold miners' roads—just beyond
La Verendrye Provincial Park into forested regions
where water is dominant domain, where an insect-plagued
moose might swim from an island and disappear again
before you have really seen it, only hearing the movement
of tree limbs snapping—my index finger
explores the map's vignettes, reminding me of
the old gods blowing new worlds from their breath
drawn in lines across latitudes.

Starting at the compass rose, I am reminded of sailors
who sought passage in the face of calamitous storms.

As my father before me, I am drawn to maps,
but I suspect it has do to with their artistry
rather than pursuit of geodata.
Charta Cosmographic's personified winds
blowing at the brink; "Here be dragons,"
our persistent but debunked myth, limits of
actualization, a position from which sailors could
precariously hold on or tumble off the edge.

Holding contours of his map, I see my father
again plummeting to his death, a vision that
paralyzes as I force myself to contemplate these
maps and charts of the Provence of Quebec on the desk
in his library in New York. Unraveling mysteries—the role
of maps in developing cosmologies—I know my father
studied Lac Yser's topography, this map with its intricate
circles and oblongs—one inside another, concentric,
displayed on walls of his home and camp,

before dropping his lines into the enigma of those clear
waters holding secretive gray trout.

Maps are also symbolizations, so poets are drawn
in like moths. In an Antoine de Fer design,
mythic forms circle Lac Yser's topography, each
paradoxically fixed in celestial motion.
Today, a comet's trajectory is traced
photographically; planimetric maps allow us
to stray from Instrastates, GPS sends signals to find
wherever Frost's country roads diverge. Emerson Sr.
must have known as he compared maps: "What lies behind us
and what lies before us are small matters compared to
what lies within us," as his namesake Ralp Waldo Emerson
wrote. From my position, with the curtains
thrown open, I can see the constellations charted, so
I roll up my father's maps, close and lock his doors;
the designs I carry contain dreams of fishing Yser's
waters and striking gold, so I hold them fast for their journey.

We search for meaning, discovering markers,
imprinting our maps with order and pattern,
our visualization for these particularities of place where
chaos of our random fall begs to reign. As I pull away,
thinking through a problem—via analogy—to which there
is no answer, this emotional mapping threatens to bring back,
as Aiken wrote, "chaos out of shape." I look, nevertheless,
at old rolls of maps beside me and drive on into night.

During the last year of his life, when he could have admitted
his wife to a nursing home in order to have a good night's sleep,
Dad could not or would not break his promise to Phyllis Marie.

When I reexperience the pain of his loss and his death, I think about the fact that he accepted the only alternative that he could bear—his own death—over abandoning his promise to her or living without her even in all the irrational, unpredictable, and sporadically frightening behaviors that were associated with AD.

She remained—until the end of his life—the sun in his planetary sphere; his life revolved around her. Yet, for my mother, her husband was the star around which she orbited until his cataclysmic fall sent her flying out of orbit.

Returning to that Mineral State

I

Something about a stone, a stone,
a stone—when my nephew and
sister-in-law laid little colored
rocks on the marbled gravestone
that marked where my brother lay,
it wasn't a tradition I knew, but one
I found comforting, so I continued
to bring him, and my mother and
father, white quartz, pink and
gray fragments cemented in breccia,
and red-veined granite from the
lakeshores of our old cabin, a place
my father and brother loved, and one
where I find myself searching for stones,
then thinking of them again, past
imploding present tense as we kids
again smash shale slabs,
peering inside the breaks,
mysteries of creatures now remote,

extinct, in those ancient days before man,
before mammal,
and we press our fingers into
indentations, feeling ridges left
by shells harboring other lives, and
it seemed, when I was young,
that a stone could talk.

II

When I met Samuel Beckett's Lucky,
I was older then but not as old as
Lucky, with his lengthy, flowing white
hair falling about his shoulders after
they had robbed the hat from his cold
head, after he had opened his mouth
and "an abode of stones" fell out,

a stone silence, an inarticulate rock,
suggesting language had no place in
saving man or woman—until I read
that young Beckett took stones home
when he was young, saving them from
wind and water, only much later in
life did he and I link stone with bone.

III

Carrying a smooth, black pebble in
my pocket for luck, I rubbed it until aching,
remembering my little brother watching
me skimming a stone until he could beat my
toss each time across the surface,
knowing my expertise had been passed down
from my father with my mother on shore.

IV

I discover I fit inside these stones
where so many others in this layered
abode have rested.
Images of stones in hollow lands
before I pass Eliot's Cathedral,
a voice urging to "take the stone
from the stone" and "wash the
stone, wash the bone."

V

This stone that could take our worry,
mark our dead, record our time, I once
again skip across open waters, watching
until all that is shown is the leaving:
a stone, a stone, a stone.

Chapter Sixteen

Her Legacy

Interiority

Mother suddenly needed a ride home
from third coast to east coast.

The funeral director, a man with a bushy
mustache and big, soft sweaty palms, said,
"Don't worry. We do this all the time."

Then I was looking out the window
at wing silvering, wondering
who else was flying in the belly of this plane,
chilled in cavity, wrapped for burial?

Even after landing, I looked
up at aircraft, considering from then on,
mothers and fathers, sons and daughters,
husbands, wives, and lovers circling
around in that other, interstitial chamber,

the one so narrowly separating living
from the dead, their allegiances no longer

to the observable, knowable world, yet here
they are among us, seemingly volitant,
embodying enigma, compelling
emotional vistas.

Regardless of what room of our big, old house you were in, there were books stacked neatly on shelves, books leaning against a wall, books under counters and in corners. Because they were ever present, I didn't really stop to think about how their presence might have influenced me and all of my siblings, but they did.

For one thing, school was not difficult for any of us. Mom read a lot, not necessarily the books I enjoy today, but she read, and seeing her reading and find pleasure in reading had an influence on her children. Whether it was purely escapism, seeking new knowledge, or a myriad of other reasons, my mother picked up a book whenever she was able to find the time, even as she reared six children. She also read to each of us when we were very young.

An early recollection begins with me holding an open book; there were pictures of chickens on the pages I flipped through, holding this precious book on my lap as I tried tracing words with my finger and saying the sounds out loud. I could not read yet, and I distinctly still feel that moment of panic rising because I had not figured out how to decode letters. I did not cry, but I absolutely knew that I should already be reading, even though I was too young to go to school.

Although my father read, too, it was my mother who subscribed to a book club, ordering new books continuously. Even when my parents were pressed to meet their bills when I was very young, Mom managed to save enough to continue to buy books.

She is the person who first took us to the public library where we got our very own library cards all those years ago. The odor of old books and papers can be accessed by memory. I searched the shelves, seeking what I knew not yet. Mom had her own ideas about what she thought I should read. She wanted to open doors for us, and she did. After our early exposure to literature, we could walk through any of the mind's rooms. Perhaps because she was never reverential about books, perhaps because they were simply part of our ordinary experience, the books in our house became part of who we are, how we conceptualized our world.

I actually know my father's favorite book because he told me without hesitating, on more than one occasion, to my persistent question: *Two Years Before the Mast* by Richard Henry Dana Jr., a book in which Dana narrates his experiences as a sailor. It was only years later that I discovered that Dana had followed his forebears into the legal profession.[1] Dana served as a United States District Attorney during the Civil War, and he died in Italy.[2] These facts did not interest me when my father first told me about them. I tried reading the book when I was little but quickly put it down. Years later, I found entrance and finished the book my father loved.

Even as all of this seems rather diversionary, I traced Dana's life and discovered multiple resemblances to my father's. He, too, had been to Italy, although during another era, World War II, and he had also been disappointed at a very late point in his legal career by clients who left him for political reasons. Although Emerson Roy Avery Sr. was careful not to mix politics and his law practice, he was affected by his son's and daughter's entrance into local politics. Emerson Jr. decided to run for the position of Cortland County judge even though he had not been in politics for very long. In fact, he was not the party's choice for the nomination, but he went on to win the primary and then the general election. Winning that election might have been good for Cortland County, but it hurt Dad's law practice. Compounded with that event, I also entered local politics at about the same time, running for the Cortland County Legislature. I discovered that no matter how you vote on an issue, you will gain enemies simply by taking a position. Neither my brother nor I intended to hurt our father or his law practice by our activism, but our political enemies became Dad's without any action on his part. He loved us and was proud of us, but I think he felt betrayed by people he considered friends, as well as clients who left his business. Still, Dad stood by his children and believed that what we were doing was right and just. The politics of the times change, and the idea that both of these men stood up for their principles against the tides of opposition speaks volumes to me now.

It was, however, in Dana's adventures at sea as a common sailor that my father connected most strongly with this author. Although a lawyer, my father never forgot his childhood, the boy growing up in poverty in the country on a small farm. He ran over the hills between Newark Valley and Maine, New York, where wild apple trees peppered the hillside. His attitude spoke to how he addressed other people, as a man of the people. It made perfect sense to him when a farmer paid his legal bill with a package of deer meat or a skinned and cleaned pheasant. Of course, that never made sense to my mother.

Phyllis Marie's favorite book would be impossible to determine because she would always give a different answer. She might have said *Little Women* at one point, but then again, she might have mentioned a murder mystery she was in the middle of reading. Her choices were eclectic, but our exposure to genres within genres came from our mother. She did, on occasion, mention Thornton Wilder, who I read while in high school but did not particularly appreciate at the time.

Recently, Jennifer Kirchoff, a friend and colleague at work, gave me a book she brought back from a teaching conference at which she was presenting. I took an extended look at the slight book and recognized that I had read Wilder's *The Bridge of San Luis Rey* when I was sixteen or seventeen, in another life. I had no intention of reading it again since there are so many great works that I have not yet read, but then I made either the mistake or had the good fortune of opening the cover, starting with the Foreword by Russell Banks, and turning to the first line of the tale in which, "the finest bridge in all Peru broke and precipitated five travelers into the gulf below."[3]

Of course, I was hooked again. I reread Wilder's thin volume but richly dense fictional account with a discerning eye, and at the end, I knew precisely why I had been given that novella. It was a reminder of what I had subconsciously known all along.

According to Russell Banks in his Foreword to a new edition of Wilder's fictional account, former British Prime Minister Tony Blair read the ending of *The Bridge of San Luis Rey* at a memorial service for those killed in the attacks on the World Trade Center in New York City.[4] I did not hear Blair's utterances, but felt the echo of them. Wilder completed his work of literature with the haunting sentences: "But soon we shall die and all memory of those five will have left the earth, and we ourselves shall be loved for a while and forgotten. But the love will have been enough."[5]

And then the line follows that I realized I had been subconsciously searching for: "Even memory is not necessary for love."[6] My mother's loss of her memory did not end love, for memory was not a prerequisite for my parent's love of each other even at the end of their lives, or of their children's love for them. Without question, part of Phyllis Marie's legacy was her love, variably fierce then quiet, in many instances confusing to her children, but she deeply loved my father, her parents, her children, her grandchildren, and her students, and love moves in multiple directions at once.

Wilder's words do not seem to exhort optimism, but they powerfully console: "There is a land of the living and a land of the dead and the bridge is love, the only survival, the only meaning."[7]

The Narrative Turn

One of the four rhetorical modes,
the Story became people who
wandered into our house through invitation
of our mother. It wasn't remarkableness
of the things she did or saw, but
the way she told them.

We knew when she broke her
arm, when she drove her father's
car, at the age of 11, through the
garage door, all the boys who fell
in love with her until she became
the murmur in my father's heart.

She repeated her life stories in a
cycle like life itself, with
tales coming up behind us
again. We thought she told
them repeatedly so that she
would never forget, but
perhaps it was so we could
never dismiss. She reshaped

our world in the narrative turn,
made us destined to seek
meaning in the province of
tales and the tellers. When we
were young, we were listeners,
before the rebellion when we
became raconteurs. Each
of her children creating allegories
we recognize, just as Tim O'Brien
said, "Stories are for eternity,
when memory is erased, when
there is nothing to remember
except the story," and we'll
recall the literature, the songs,
the history that make us human.

Phyllis was a storyteller. We knew her stories almost as well as she did because she told them so often, sometimes revealing a new detail here and there. It was not hard to imagine her as a little girl or a pretty, headstrong teenager. We could visualize her arm in a cast when she fell skating, later sitting at her desk in third grade, trying to write with her left hand as her teacher looked on disapprovingly at the slant of her penmanship. Admittedly, we tired of her stories when we were young. It was as if she was afraid that she would forget them, so she told and retold each one, crafting the scene from details she could pull from recollection.

Looking back in order to see where I am now, it almost seemed as if my mother could foresee her disease and her own end like Aureliano Babilonia, reading the parchments that predicted his death and the destruction of his town in Gabriel García Márquez's novel *One Hundred Years of Solitude*: "Before reaching the final line, however, he had already understood that he would never leave that room, for it was foreseen that the city of mirrors (or mirages) would be wiped out by the wind and exiled from the memory of men . . ."[8]

And I think of García Márquez because he was a supreme storyteller—better than my mother. Yet, I'd like to believe that had they met my mother would have charmed him, or at least told him a few tales of her own.

Growing up in my parents' house, I was engulfed by photo albums, reels of films from the early days of home movies, and family pictures in frames. There were dresser drawers stuffed with old, loose photos, waiting for homes. As far back as I can call to mind, I was in the middle of the history of my family, and my mother was the keeper of those stories, the collector of our archives, telling us the tales of lightning striking first a tree and then a man in her backyard, of her adventure driving a car and crashing it through a garage door when she was eleven, of my father's older brother Robert who was killed in the war, trying desperately to make it to the shore in the midst of strafing gunfire and bombs.

My mother got my father to talk about his war experiences, and she encouraged him to share these stories with my nephew who later created a tape of their conversations. Emerson Sr. did not want to talk about the war, but he had shared all of these experiences with my mother who told the tales to us.

It was from my mother that we first learned that my father held a narrative that would affect how he viewed the rest of his life, how he looked at the world from that point forward. Only much later, would my father add a few details we had never heard before: of the day he got a terrible cold, maybe strep throat, and it turned out to be the greatest fortune for him to be sick, because he was scheduled for a routine flyover while in Northern Africa with his crew.

Of course, this was during World War II, and he was but seventeen years old—having lied about his age in order to serve his country. His crew members were his friends, the young guys he had trained with before setting off for Europe first and then Africa, but he was sick, so sick that when he came out with watery eyes and an inaudible voice, the rest of the guys on the mission told him to go back to base. Told him that he wasn't needed on this trip; it would be an unremarkable flight in which they were simply testing equipment and doing an aerial survey.

After much protesting, Emerson Roy finally acquiesced and returned to his bunk to spend a miserable afternoon, sleeping fitfully in a fever. Only a few hours later, however, he was awakened and told that his plane carrying his friends and fellow farm boys went down. They were all dead. In that instant, his life was forever changed.

In some respects, that event shaped his view, his great empathy for others, his compassion, his generosity, his kindness, and his inherent belief that he was a lucky man. It also hinted at his incautious optimism and partially explained one of his favorite phrases: "Most people are basically good." I never quite agreed with him on that analysis of humanity, but I liked the fact that he held it so closely. It was a lovely way to look at the world. My father went on and lived a full life in which he helped many people, but we would never have known this story—because of his recalcitrance—if not for my mother.

I wonder if my mother had secrets. She must have. She talked about macrocosms and microcosms, and there were no taboo subjects, although she was delicate how she phrased certain topics. Phyllis could describe the most brutal exchange between human beings and never use a crude word.

Her legacy lays with her stories, her children, her grandchildren, her great-grandson, and her many students who have grown up and moved on in life. Phyllis Marie was dynamic, energetic, driven, artistic, lovely, lonely in a house filled with kids, tough to argue with, sometimes just difficult, politically and socially conscious, opinionated, compassionate and impassioned, and so much more.

She was a teacher even before she entered her elementary classrooms. As far back as I have a memory, she was teaching someone about what she knew. She was a chronicler of tales and life itself. Framing life, in some respects, as story, she gave us the structure within which we would navigate that course.

At our mother's funeral, my youngest brother Larry stood up and offered a tribute to Phyllis Marie Unold Avery. He also said in front of that gathering that, "everything I am, I owe to my mother." As he spoke, I looked around and saw the surprise on some people's faces. Emerson had been such a force in all of our lives, and I knew how dearly my youngest brother loved our father, but my brother was speaking honestly and from the heart; it made sense to me. Even in her mercurial moods, our mother was the person most responsible for shaping our lives. She was the parent who got up in the night and tended to us during our many illnesses; she was the one who read to us, she was the primary disciplinarian, and she was the one who could use a line that cut deeply because she knew each of us so well.

I knew already—before my mother's illness and death— that I was a writer and a teacher because Phyllis Marie was my mother. Like my mother, I am not a historian recording the facts precisely in the order in which they occurred, but I am a narrator who seeks out the emotional resonance of a tale to relate it once again, weaving in the surfaces as well as the depths only hinted at in the frame. Even as I fought against it, I became my mother's daughter.

Her legacy was not—would not be—this disease. Phyllis Marie Unold Avery told us stories. She recited them all and thought we should know, so as to never forget. Because I cannot restore, it is my promise to her that for as long as I am able, I will recognize, restory, and remember.

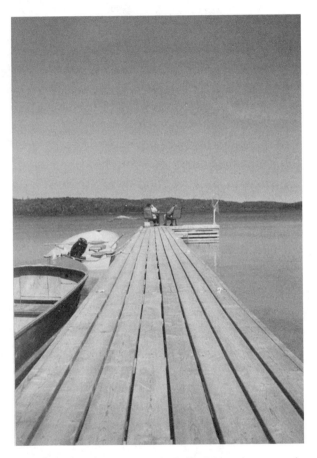

Figure 5. Emerson Roy Avery Sr. and Phyllis Marie Avery are shown together in a brief moment of peace in this photo on their last trip to their camp in Quebec, Canada.

Chapter Seventeen

Shadows

Tattooed

Waiting to be deciphered by
Madame Sosostris or Sibyl,
we wear our stories,
embedded in lines of our smiles,
the curve of our backs, the way
we hold a pen, scars
over our hearts,
the changing tenor of a
once familiar voice.
Only a handful ever
practice and become
proficient at reading
the invisible.

Even after the deaths of people we love, we are still with them in our struggles and our joys. Mom and Dad are present in my life and they will continue to be, but their presence lies in an isolated gesture I recognize, an expression on my face that calls up the image of my mother. I hear echoes of my father's footsteps when I walk to the end of the dock at his camp in Quebec.

I hear his voice in my head when I hold my fingertip to the monofilament line, coaxing the fish beneath those deep waters. Standing in my classroom, I occasionally hear my mother's words come out of my mouth. I am still surprised.

Sometimes it's a song on the radio in the car, and I am riding with them on the way to other journeys. But I miss them, and I know they would have loved meeting their great-grand-children. "Truman looks kind of like your father," someone said; I know I look like my mother.

As I move into a new period and try to shift the past into the past, I am again startled. One day, some period after her death, I walked up the back stairs to an antique shop and found not antiquity but yesterday, found objects belonging to my mother that never should have been in that dusty little room. I might have cried or yelled, but instead I held them up, purchased the tea set, and then took them home.

Ornament

The gold rim of the tea set mirrors the gilt edge of my
writing journal's page.
There on my dining table, the salt shakers stand tall,
pairing off against the triad,
the teapot all opaque alabaster ringed with gold, sug-
gesting opulence.
The sugar and creamer promise a supporting cast. I
stare at my find,
recalling my pursuit of serendipity in the anarchy of a
second-story junk shop,
picking through the discarded, temporal remnants, care-
fully winding my way
so as not to break the fragile lives poised for a fall.

I'm looking for a mirror, just a fragment of reflective
  glass
that will hang on the camp's south wall, Lac Yser's
  doppelgänger.
The mirrors are pricey, old wood, musty and aberrant,
precariously surrounding beveled glass. I find one without a price tag.
"How much for this mirror?" "Oh, that's very old,
  very fine, but
I could . . . my best price . . . I couldn't go lower
  than $285." "No.
Thank you." I turn away ready to leave when I spot
  an unframed,
thick beauty marred by use, losing her silvering,
  appearing stippled,
but the size and rustic charm of the chipped edging
  attract my attention.
I lean close, examine the price tag, and triumphantly
  hoist my Venus
up from the floor where it was leaning.

It is only when I turn to go that I recognize the ala-
  baster china.
It stops me.
I remember these characters from another life:
A little girl dusting the ceramics in the hutch when her
  mother gasps.

"Be careful with those!" Fragments.
Memories stored in rooms I seldom visit. But how?
I lay down the prized mirror and examine the tea set.
  "Do you know

where this set came from?" "Well, it's been here some
   time, at least a year."
"When my father died, we had to sell all of their possessions. It looks like hers."
I do not tell her about my mother's Alzheimer's.
She shifts position."The name?" I give her their names
   and date of the sale.

"Yes. Yes," she says, leafing through the registry at her
   worn desk.
 "What could you sell this set for?" I try not to sound
   desperate,
already knowing I will buy back my mother's china.
 I help her wrap each piece in thick, white blanketing
   paper, the tops first,
trying not to show the deluge of emotions streaming.

At home again, I uncover the set, carefully placing it
   on the oak table
that seems too humble for these gifts. I consider the
   inherent absurdity of buying back
what was once my mother's, and I measured how
   fiercely I wanted her back
as I stared at the alabaster and gold face of her tea set.

After the Fall

After the fall
and the pneumonia,
after the disease
and the funerals,
after the filling out of papers
and more papers

After the loss upon loss
upon loss spoken as onslaught,

After all this,
there is a tiny, red,
beaded coin purse
locked away in a safe deposit
box.

Inside, neatly folded,
a two-dollar bill is inscribed.
Written in red ink
is a date and the words,
"love you more than—"

After all this,
there is still mystery.

Appendix A

Turning to the Web

There are numerous clinical trials—by the National Institute on Aging—taking place in the United States that may produce the kind of results whereby people with a predisposition toward Alzheimer's may take steps or medicines to help extend the period before onset.[1] We are not there yet, but there is reason to be hopeful.

The more that is learned about the pathosis, the greater the possibility that specific medications may be developed and sold that could either ward off the onset of the disease entirely or prolong it to such an extent that it would not be a factor in life decisions.

Clinical trials are taking place that examine a number of factors on how Alzheimer's progresses. Vitamin D appears to be positively linked to either preventing or slowing the progress of the disorder. According to Professor Tetsuya Terasaki in his paper published in BioMed Central, an open access journal, *Fluids and Barriers of the CNS*, Alzheimer's research "shows that removal of amyloid ß from the brain depends on vitamin D and also on an age-related alteration in the production of transporter proteins which move amyloid ß in and out of the brain."[2]

Although the study dealt with vitamin D in the brains of mice, the research appears promising: Professor Terasaki stated,

"Vitamin D appears to increase transport of amyloid ß across the blood brain barrier (BBB) by regulating protein expression, via the vitamin D receptor, and also by regulating cell signaling via the MEK pathway. These results lead the way towards new therapeutic targets in the search for prevention of Alzheimer's disease."[3]

The following are some websites for reliable, updated, factual, and helpful information:

- A Place for Living, Trusted Senior Living Advisors, and A Place for Mom, Inc., 2000–2013. http://www.aplaceformom.com/.

- This website helps you navigate through the choices of assisted living options for people with Alzheimer's disease. You can enter your location, and the search engine will filter through the choices and find those closest to you.

- BioMed Central is an "open access publisher" of hundreds of medical and scientific journals that feature some of the latest research in medicine. A quick search, using the website's search window, reveals over 160 of the latest articles on new research and findings related to AD. http://www. biomedcentral.com/journals.

- Healthy Place, America's Mental Health Channel website has a great deal of information, including specifics on the typically prescribed medications for people with Alzheimer's. The website is easy to navigate with a table of contents on the homepage: http://www.healthyplace.com/alzheimers/.

- Ina Jaffe reports on, discusses, and writes about a program that is helping caregivers of those with Alzheimer's on NPR's *All Things Considered*. You can listen to the story or download the transcript from NPR's website at: http://www.npr.org/2013/01/08/168890934/workshops-help-families-grappling-with-alzheimers-home-care.

- The Alzheimer's Association website breaks down the facts from the fiction, provides information about warning signs, medications, treatments, and so on. In addition, this invaluable web resource has a search page to help find health care providers in your area: http://www.alz.org/index.asp.

- The Alzheimer's Foundation of America website offers a tremendous amount of information, including a media center page where events centered on Alzheimer's research and awareness are being held: www.alzfdn.org.

- The American Health Assistance Foundation's website has a separate page on Alzheimer's resources that includes legal and financial assistance information, as well as specifics on health care providers, according to city addresses. This website also has a page devoted to books that are helpful to caregivers: www.ahaf.org.

- The U.S. government National Institutes of Health sites, specifically the National Institute on Aging: http://www.nia.nih.gov/Alzheimers/.

- WebMD.com has a great deal of information, particularly about symptoms, including early symptoms of the disease. It also has a page on "brain foods" that help concentration. I have been eating more berries, avocados, and drinking more coffee ever since: www.webmd.com/alzheimers.

Appendix B

Texts on the Subject

Alzheimer's has been in the media spotlight in recent years with nonfiction books for caregivers published, poems written, movies released, and memoirs penned about people battling this deadly illness that robs memories and our sense of who we are and how we are connected. More medical and scientific information should eventually lead to better understanding of the disease as well as how to help both those who have the disease and those who serve as caregivers.

- *Beyond Alzheimer's: How to Avoid the Modern Epidemic of Dementia* by Scott D. Mendelson, MD, PhD, M. Evans and Company, an Imprint of Rowman & Littlefield Publishers, 2009.

- Maria Shriver wrote the book *What's Happening to Grandpa* about her father—the statesman, vice presidential candidate, and founder of the Jobs Corps, Head Start, and one of the leaders in helping to create the Peace Corps—(Robert) Sargent Shriver Jr. and the Alzheimer's that altered their lives before he died in January 2011. Her book is written for children to help them understand the dramatic changes that the disease wrests.

- *The 36-Hour Day: A Family Guide to Caring for Persons Who Have Alzheimer Disease, Related Dementias, and Memory Loss* (5th ed.), by Nancy L. Mace, MA, and Peter V. Rabins, MD, MPH, is simply one of the most helpful texts you can get on this subject.

- *The Alzheimer's Action Plan: The Experts' Guide to the Best Diagnosis and Treatment for Memory Problems* by P. Murali Doraiswamy, MD, Lisa P. Gwyther, MSW, Tina Adler is thorough, particularly from the standpoint of early diagnosis and treatment options.

- *Validation Breakthrough: Simple Techniques for Communicating with People with Alzheimer's-Type Dementia*, 3rd ed., by Naomi Feil, Vicki de Klerk-Rubin, published by Health Professions Press, 2012. The first edition was published in 1993. This text was one that I discovered only after going through trial and painful error with my mother. I only wish I had come across this book much earlier.

Index of Poems

Notes

Acknowledgments

1. Vladimir Nabokov, *Speak, Memory* (New York: Random House, 1947, 1948, 1951, 1967), 8.

A Note on the Title

1. Vladimir Nabokov, Lolita, 50th Anniversary ed., 2nd Vintage Int. ed., June, 1997 (New York: Random House, 1955, 1995).

2. Orhan Pamuk, *Other Colors*, trans. Maureen Freely (Toronto: Alfred A. Knopf, 2007), 157.

Introduction: After the Fall

1. U.S. National Institutes of Health, U.S. government, updated daily, accessed February 12, 2012, www.nia.nih.gov/Alzheimers.

2. James Joyce, *Ulysses*, Everyman's Library ed. (New York: Knopf Doubleday, [1922]1997),

Chapter One: Uncertainty

1. Howard Nemerov, "The Human Condition," *Collected Poems of Howard Nemerov* (Chicago: University of Chicago Press, 1981).

2. *About Alzheimer's Disease: Alzheimer's Basic.* National Institute on Aging, U.S. Department of Health and Human Services, updated daily, accessed January, 2012, http://www.nia.nih.gov/ alzheimers/topics/alzheimers-basics.

3. *About Alzheimer's Disease.*National Institute on Aging. 4. William Shakespeare, *Macbeth*, act V, scene I, 1, 19.

5. Nabokov, *Speak, Memory*, 33.

Chapter Two: Why Now? Why My Family?

1. Emery University, Alzheimer's Disease Research Center,

2. Alzheimer Europe, updated November 9, 2012, accessed December 27, 2012, http://www.alzheimer-europe.org/News/Dementia-in-Society/Monday-09-July-2012-Gabriel-Garcia-Marquez-can-no-longer-write-due-to-dementia.

3. "Garcia Marquez Foundation Refutes Dementia Claim," American Free Press, July 9, 2012, accessed March 11, 2012, http://www.google.com/hostednews/afp/article.

4. Alzheimer's Overview, Complete Wellness Center, HealthAtoZ.com, Medical Network Inc., updated June 7, 2007, accessed March 11, 2012, 1999–2005, http://cerner.healthatoz.com/Atoz/dc/caz/neur/alzh/alzunder.asp.

5. "Battling Alzheimer's Disease," November 30, 2012, Clarity Digital Group, accessed March 11, 2012, 2006–2013, Examiner.com, http://www.examiner.com/article.

6. Ibid.

Chapter Four: Mistaken Identities

1. Oliver Sacks, *The Man Who Mistook His Wife for a Hat: And Other Clinical*, First Touchstone ed. (New York: Touchstone, Simon & Schuster, 1998).

2. Ibid.

3. Orhan Pamuk, *Silent House*, trans. Robert Finn, Borzoi Books (New York: Alfred A. Knopf, trans. 2012), 332.

Chapter Six: You Look Like Your Mother

1. Mental Health Forum, last modified 2013, date accessed March 9, 2012, http:www.mentalhealthforum.net/forum/.
2. Nabokov, *Speak, Memory*, 25–26.

Chapter Nine: Icebergs in Paradise

1. Elizabeth Luke, "The Affliction," ESM Central Schools, unpublished paper, 2013.
2. Jonah Lehrer, "The Forgetting Pill Erases Painful Memories Forever," February 17, 2012, *Wired*, Conde Nast, March, 2012, http://www.wired.com/magazine/2012/02/ff_forgettingpill/.
3. Ibid.

Chapter Twelve: Did You See The Notebook?

1. *The Notebook film script*, Drew's Script-O-Rama, movie based on the Nicholas Sparks book, accessed February 2012, www.script-o-rama.com.
2. Ibid.

Chapter Fourteen: Managing in a Nursing Home or Assisted Living Facility

1. Maira Kalman, *The Principles of Uncertainty* (New York: Penguin Group, 2007).

Chapter Fifteen: Collecting Memories

1. Therese A. Rando, "Bereaved Parents: Particular Difficulties, Unique Factors, and Treatment Issues," *Social Work* 30, no. 1, (1985): 20.

2. Atwood, Margaret, "Happy Endings," Onondaga Community College, January 30, 2013 http://occonline.occ.cccd.edu/online/swells/Happy%20Endings.pdf.

Chapter Sixteen: Her Legacy

1. Richard Henry Dana, *Two Years Before the Mast and Twenty-Four Years After*, 63rd printing, 1969 (P. F. Collier & Son).
2. Charles Francis Adams, *Richard Henry Dana*, Harvard College Library, 3rd ed. (Boston and New York: Houghton Mifflin, 1891).
3. Thornton Wilder, *The Bridge of San Luis Rey*, Perennial Classics, 2003, Foreword and Afterword (New York: Perennial, imprint of HarperCollins Publishers), 5.
4. Russell Banks, Foreword, *The Bridge of San Luis Rey* by Thornton Wilder, xvi.
5. Thornton Wilder, *The Bridge of San Luis Rey*, First Perennial Classics, (New York: Perennial, imprint of HarperCollins Publishers [1955]2003), 107.
6. Ibid.
7. Ibid.
8. Gabriel Garcia Marquez, *One Hundred Years of Solitude*, Perennial Classics ed., 1998 (New York: HarperCollins), 447–448.

Appendix A: Turning to the Web

1. National Institute on Aging, U.S. government, U.S. Department of Health and Human Services, updated daily, ww.nia.nih.gov/alzheimers.
2. Tetsuya Terasaki, "Advances in Research into Alzheimer's Disease: Transporter Proteins at the Blood CSF Barrier and Vitamin D May Help Prevent Amyloid ß Build Up in the Brain," BioMedCentral, July 8, 2011, http://www.biomedcentral.com/presscenter/pressreleases/20110708.
3. Ibid.

About the Author

Nancy Avery Dafoe is a published writer and poet, in addition to being an English educator working and living in Central New York. Her book *Breaking Open the Box: A Guide for Creative Techniques to Improve Academic Writing and Generate Critical Thinking* was published in March 2013. A companion book, *Writing Creatively: A Guided Journal to Using Literary Devices*, was published by Rowman & Littlefield Education in February 2014. Excerpts from Dafoe's plays are included in the anthology *Lost Orchard*, edited by Jo Pitkin, published by SUNY Press in January 2014. Her fiction and poetry have won numerous awards, including first place in the New Century Writer and Soul-Making Literary contests, and her work has appeared in a number of literary magazines and publications. *An Iceberg in Paradise: A Passage Through Alzheimer's* was a finalist in the 2013 William Faulkner/William Wisdom Creative Writing competition, nonfiction category.

She has taught in a variety of settings, including high school and college. Prior to teaching, Dafoe worked as a journalist and in the field of public relations.

Dafoe currently resides in Homer, New York, with her husband Daniel, son Blaise, and dog Bogart.